Low Carb Diet Cookbook

Diet for Beginners

The Ultimate Beginners Diet to Low Carb

By Logan Thomas

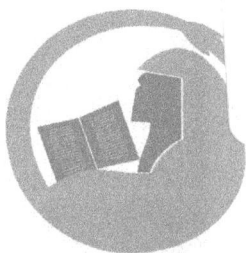

EFFINGO
Publishing

Download another book for Free

We want to thank you for purchasing this book and offer you another book (just as long and valuable as this book), "Health & Fitness Mistakes You Don't Know You're Making", completely free.

Visit the link below to sign up and receive it:

www.effingopublishing.com/gift

In this book, we will break down the most common health & fitness mistakes, you are probably committing right now, and will reveal how you can easily get in the best shape of your life!

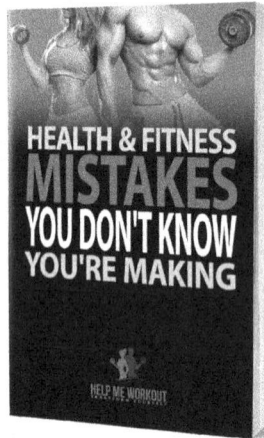

In addition to this valuable gift, you will also have an opportunity to get our new books for free, enter giveaways, and receive other valuable emails from us. Again, visit the link to sign up:

www.effingopublishing.com/gift

Table of Contents

INTRODUCTION

Before you get started, I recommend you <u>joining our</u> <u>email newsletter</u> to receive updates on any upcoming new book releases or promotions. You can sign up for free, and as a bonus, you will receive a gift. Our *"Health & Fitness Mistakes You Don't Know You're Making"* book! This book has been written to demystify, expose the top do's and don'ts and to finally equip you with the information you need to get in the best shape of your life. Due to the overwhelming amount of misinformation and lies told by magazines and self-proclaimed "gurus," it's becoming harder and harder to get reliable information to get in shape. As opposed to having to go through dozens of biased, unreliable, and untrustworthy sources to get your health & fitness information. Everything you need to help you has been broken down in this book for you to easily follow and to immediately get results to achieve your desired fitness goals in the shortest amount of time.

Once again, to join our free email newsletter and to receive a free copy of this valuable book, please visit the link and sign up now: <u>www.effingopublishing.com/gift.</u>

What to Eat and What to avoid

As people with cravings from time to time, we tend to go to a quicker solution for food preparations of fast foods like burgers, pizzas, and sometimes other homemade meals that found its way to our lives due to convenience. Disregarding our health, we settle for comfort but not to worry. There is a solution! And it is just as convenient as the fast foods and as easy to get accustomed to.

Wheat has been finding its way to our plates since breakfast, through lunch, and finally dinner. As it helps keeps our tummy full, it also keeps us from losing weight and keeping fit. Bread as the general of all carbohydrates-related foods must be avoided. Fortunately, there is a suitable replacement, and it is teff. If you have heard of quinoa (An alternative of rice, pasta), teff has 20% more nutrients that promote weight loss, like high fiber, and it was also reported that teff has more proteins than quinoa. Although there are other re-placements for bread (different kinds), teff is the most efficient.

Another critical thing I would like to add is in the fruit section. Picture this, Sandra and Emily are friends from high school and are having a reunion with the rest of her classmates. Sandra has some belly fat she would like to get rid of. They both want to eat outside. Sandra loves fruits, so she always orders juice. The reunion is in 2 weeks, and Sandra would like to make the most of it. Unfortunately, instead of losing weight, she gains a pound or two. How might you ask? Because most of the time, restaurants and cafes like to put a little more sugar and stuff to make their drinks more pleasing and enslave your taste buds. You do not want to be that person whose motivation is lost due to some rudimentary decisions. That is why we are here to help YOU. Fruits like oranges, kiwi (raw with no sugar) are so low in calories that the body burns more calories on the regular. There are also some vegetables that do a better job in terms of metabolism and weight loss than some fruits.

Vegetables, the food section mostly ignored in popular culture (as kids) but will go running towards it after puberty (and even then we'll have walls to climb). Vegetables like cabbage, promote a feeling of having a full stomach and promotes faster waste removal. It's a two in one package deal! On the other side, some carrots help the liver in bile secretion (in other words, weight loss).

Health Benefits and Risks

Once upon a time, in the Garden of Eden, a man and a woman had the advantage of having all the kinds of food within a walk-and-pluck distance. They were told that all the foods that they saw were right for them (except for that one tree, disregard it for now). Nowadays, as beneficial as they are, some foods can cause more damage if taken beyond limited usage.

Name one that can make you it's murder and widower (at the same time). Onions. We mostly eat them with fried foods and just this once I will say that it's OK. Onions are useful for reducing depression, high in vitamins; there is even some report of it that it prevents cancer. But when taking too much of it, it can cause stomach problems like bloating, cramps, even ulcers. It is said that fruits and vegetables are high in their nutrients when taken raw. In this case, I think it's OK to let some of the nutrients go through a process of cooking.

Pineapples as effective as they are; they could also be damaging. Taking too much of pineapples could lead to consequences such as diarrhea, nausea, vomiting, abdominal pain, or heartburn. This is because of its high amount of Vitamin C.

Here we are going to provide you 50+ Proven Fat Burn Low Carb Weight Loss Recipes, which includes breakfast, lunch, dinner, and night meals. You can follow it well.

RECIPES FOR BREAKFAST

Bacon, Egg, And Cheese Roll up

Ingredients:

- 6 large eggs
- 2 tablespoon milk
- ¼ garlic powder
- Kosher salt
- Freshly ground black pepper
- 1 tablespoon butter
- 1 tablespoon finely chopped chives
- 12 slices bacon
- 2 cups of shredded cheddar

How to Make:

1. Mix eggs, milk, garlic powder salt, and pepper in a large bowl.

2. Melt butter in the frying pan (medium heat), add the mix to the pan and stir for 3 minutes.

3. Lay the bacon strips on a plate. Sprinkle bottom parts of bacon with cheddar and top parts with a spoonful of the scrambled mix. Roll them.

4. Place the rolls on the frying pan. Cook until all sides become crispy.

Nutrition Facts:

- Per serving: 389 Calories

- 26.3 grams of Total Fat
- 10.6 grams of Saturated Fat
- 330 milligrams of Cholesterol
- 1172 milligrams of Sodium
- 2.6 grams of Total Carbohydrate
- 0.1 gram of Dietary Fibre
- 1.3 grams of Sugars
- 34.1 grams of Protein
- Vitamin D 141%
- Calcium 22%
- Iron 11%
- Potassium 7%

Ham & Cheese Egg Cups

Ingredients:

- Cooking spray for pan
- 12 slices ham
- 1 cup shredded cheddar
- 12 large eggs
- Kosher Salt
- Freshly ground black pepper
- Chopped fresh parsley, for garnish
- 12-cup muffin tin

How to Make:

1. Before starting, heat the oven to 400 degrees Fahrenheit.
2. Spray a 12-cup muffin tin with the cooking spray.
3. Place the slices of ham on each muffin tin cup to form a cup. Sprinkle cheddar and crack an egg into each cup. Add salt and pepper.
4. Put in the oven for 12 to 15 minutes.
5. Serve the dish with the chopped fresh parsley to your liking.

Nutrition Facts:

- Per serving: 340 calories
- 12 grams of protein
- 10 grams of carbohydrates
- 7 grams of fiber

- 1 gram of sugar
- 30 grams of fat
- 9 grams of saturated fat
- 240 milligrams of sodium

Magic Low-Carb Waffles

Ingredients:

- 6 large eggs
- 2 bananas mashed
- 2 tablespoons unsweetened almond butter
- Kosher salt
- ½ tablespoons ground cinnamon
- Cooking spray
- ½ tablespoon coconut butter
- ½ tablespoon almond butter
- ¼ banana, sliced
- ½ tablespoon chopped walnuts
- 1 tablespoon maple syrup or coconut nectar
- Waffle iron
- Batter (as needed)

How to Make

1. Before starting, heat waffle iron.

2. Mix the eggs, bananas, almond butter, whole-wheat flour, cinnamon, and salt.

3. Spray waffle iron with Cooking Spray.

4. Add batter and cook until golden.

5. Put waffles in the fridge in a resealable container and serve with desired toppings (coconut butter, walnuts, maple syrup, coconut nectar).

Nutrition Facts

- Per serving: 248 calories
- Total Fat 14.4 grams
- Saturated Fat 3.2 grams
- Cholesterol 279 milligrams
- Sodium 146 milligrams
- Total Carbohydrate 20.2 grams
- Dietary Fibre 3.2 grams
- Total Sugars 11.3 grams
- Protein 12.5 grams
- Vitamin C 26 micrograms
- Calcium 58 milligrams
- Iron 4 milligrams
- Potassium 406 milligrams

Bacon Weave Breakfast Tacos

Ingredients:

- 16 slices bacon
- Freshly ground black pepper
- 6 large eggs
- 1 tablespoon whole milk
- 1 tablespoon butter
- Kosher salt
- 2 tablespoons chopped chives
- ¼ shredded Monterey jack
- 1 avocado
- Hot sauce

How to Make:

1. Before starting, Heat oven to 400 degrees Fahrenheit and place an aluminum foil.

2. Make bacon take the shapes of squares (4 slices of bacon each).

3. Add pepper to bacon squares.

4. Place the 3 squared slices of bacon in the oven and bake for 30–35 minutes until crispy

5. Mix eggs with milk in a bowl.

6. Melt butter in a skillet (bowl-shaped frying pan) then pour in the milk and egg mixture

7. Mix with a spatula carefully.

8. After the eggs are cooked, add salt and pepper.

9. After 30–35 minutes have passed, use a knife to carve the slices of bacon to give them round-like shapes.

10. After all other steps are done, place the scrambled eggs inside the bacon (3 of them). Sprinkle cheese, add a few slices of avocado, and hot sauce as topping.

Nutrition Facts:

- Per serving: 390 calories

- 24 grams of protein

- 4 grams of carbohydrates

- 2 grams of fiber

- 1 gram of sugar

- 31 grams of fat

- 11 grams of saturated fat

- 720 milligrams of sodium

Cauliflower Benedict

Ingredients:

- ½ head cauliflower
- 6 large eggs
- 1 cup of shredded cheddar
- Pinch of cornstarch
- Kosher salt
- Freshly grounded pepper
- 1 tablespoon extra-virgin olive oil
- A squeeze of lemon juice
- 1 stick butter melted
- Pinch of cayenne pepper
- 2 slices of bacon
- Paprika
- Chives

How to Make:

1. Before starting, chop chives and prepare warm paprika.
2. Shred the cauliflower on a box grater (shredder box).
3. Add and mix the shredded cauliflower and 1 egg and to a bowl.
4. Add cheddar and cornstarch and season with salt.
5. Heat the oil in a large skillet in a temperature of medium-high heat.

6. Add a spoonful of the cauliflower egg mixture and shape into patties (repeat until the bowl is empty).

7. Cook the cauliflower egg mixture until it is crispy with a color of brown:5 minutes cooking one side, then flip and cook the other side for 5 minutes as well.

8. Boil water in a sauce-pan, then reduce the heat to simmer.

9. While Stirring the water to add 1 egg (not cracked) to get a right mix. Let it cook for 3 minutes

10. Afterward, place the egg on a plate, paper towel, or on any other food-placing material that seems convenient to you. (Repeat process for 1 more egg).

11. With the remaining water in the saucepan, make a hollandaise: remove two inches of water and reduce the temperature of heat to a low simmer.

12. Place a heatproof bowl on the saucepan.

13. Add 4 egg yolks and lemon juice and mix them.

14. Add butter and stir in steady motion until a combined solution is formed, then add salt and cayenne.

15. Serve the cauliflower hash brown patties with toppings of bacon, boiled eggs, and the hollandaise with sides chopped chives and paprika.

Nutrition Facts:

- Per serving: 683 calories

- 57 grams of fat

- 8 grams of Carbohydrates

- 2 grams of Fibre

- 35 grams of Protein

Crustless Quiche

Ingredients:

- 1 tablespoon of butter
- 8 ounces of cremini mushrooms, thinly sliced
- 1 shallot
- 2 cups of loosely packed spinach
- Kosher salt
- Freshly ground black pepper
- 8 large eggs
- ¼ cups of whole milk
- ¼ cups of oil-packed sun-dried tomatoes, chopped
- Freshly grated Parmesan

How to Make:

1. Before starting, Heat oven to 375 degrees Fahrenheit.
2. Melt butter in a skillet in medium heat.
3. Add mushrooms to the skillet and let it cook (not mixed) for 2 minutes.
4. Now start stirring the mushrooms in the skillet for 5 to 6 minutes until mushrooms are tender and golden.
5. Add shallot and cook until the scent of fragrant.
6. Add spinach and cook 1 minute more after wilting.
7. Add salt and pepper.
8. Mix eggs, milk, tomatoes, and Parmesan in a bowl
9. Put the mushroom mixture in the bowl and add salt and pepper again.

10. Vierta todo en un plato para pastel de 8 a 9 pulgadas y hornee hasta que los huevos estén cocidos de 18 a 20 minutos.

11. Afterward, let it cool (3 minutes recommended), and it's ready to be served.

Nutrition Facts

- Per Serving: 217.6 calories
- 15.1 gram of Fat
- 7.5 gram of Saturated Fat
- 0.7 gram of Polyunsaturated Fat
- 3 grams of Monounsaturated Fat
- 184.6 milligrams of cholesterol
- 597 milligrams of Sodium
- 52.6 milligrams of Potassium
- 3.7 grams of Total Carbohydrate
- 0.4 gram of Dietary Fibre
- 1.6 grams of Sugars
- 17.1 grams of Protein
- Vitamin A 19%
- Vitamin B-12 4.5%
- Vitamin B-6 2.4%
- Vitamin C 9.2%
- Vitamin D 6.9%
- Vitamin E 2.4%
- Calcium 25.1%

- Copper 0.5%
- Folate 4.7%
- Iron 4.2%
- Magnesium 0.4%
- Niacin 0.0%
- Pantothenic Acid 4.1%
- Phosphorus 5.8%
- Riboflavin 4.9%
- Selenium 10.1 %
- Thiamin 1.7%
- Zinc 2.1%

Sheet Pan Brussels Sprout

Ingredients:

- 2 pounds of Brussels sprouts
- 6 slices bacon
- 2 tablespoons of buffalo sauce plus more for serving
- ½ tablespoon of garlic powder
- Pinch of salt
- Kosher salt
- Freshly ground black pepper
- 6 large Free-range eggs (eggs from hens that are permitted outdoor privileges, has health benefits)
- Freshly chopped chives

How to Make:

- Before Starting, Heat oven to 425 degrees Fahrenheit.
- Put Brussels sprouts, bacon, oil, buffalo sauce, garlic powder, and red pepper flakes in a large bowl.
- Bake in the oven for 15 minutes (until bacon is crispy and Brussels sprouts are tender)
- Make 6 nest-like circles emptying the centers, then add 1 egg to each nest, then add salt and pepper.
- Bake the eggs for 8 to 10 minutes.
- Serve with garnished chives and buffalo sauce.

Nutrition Facts:

- Calories: 113

- 6.9 grams of Fat
- 6.8 grams of Carbohydrates
- 7.9 grams of Protein

Best-Ever Shakshuka

Ingredients:

- 1 tablespoon olive oil
- ½ peeled and diced onion
- 1 minced clove garlic
- 1 seeded and chopped bell pepper
- 4 cups of ripe diced tomatoes / 2 cans 14 ounces of diced tomatoes
- 2 tablespoons of tomato paste
- 1 teaspoon of milk chili powder
- 1 teaspoon cumin
- 1 teaspoon paprika
- Pinch of cayenne pepper (option to add more for taste)
- Pinch of sugar (keep low to avoid carbs)
- Salt and pepper
- 6 eggs
- ½ tablespoon fresh chopped parsley (option to decorate)

How to Make:

1. Before starting, Heat large skillet on medium heat.
2. Slowly warm olive oil in the pan/skillet).
3. Add onion and cook until the onion softens.
4. Add garlic and continue to cook until there is a change in the scent.

5. Add the bell pepper and cook for 5 to 7 minutes over medium heat until it softens.

6. Add tomato paste and diced tomatoes to the pan. Stir until they blend.

7. Add spices and sugar, then stir for 5 to 7 minutes until it simmers

8. Add any optional extras at this stage to determine the taste.

9. Add eggs in different places of the dish (directly without beating or mixing it with the mixture in the pan).

10. Simmer for 10 to 15 minutes. Note: Make sure the sauce doesn't reduce too much.

11. (Optional) Let it run some more so the mixture can solidify.

Instant Pot Frittata

Ingredients:

- 6 eggs
- ½ teaspoon fine sea salt
- Black pepper (grinds)
- 8 ounces of chopped broccoli florets
- 3 chopped green onions,
- 2 ounces of shredded cheddar cheese
- 1 cup of water
- Cooking Spray
- Instant Pot

How to Make:

1. Mix eggs, salt, black pepper, then add chopped broccoli, green onions, and cheddar.

2. Spray a 7-inch pan, then add the mixture into it.

3. Pour the water (1 cup) into an instant pot and place a trivet over that to keep the pan above the water.

4. Place the pan with the frittata mixture on top of the trivet and secure the lid, then use the pressure cook or manual button on your machine to cook at high pressure for 10 minutes.

5. Afterward, let it release the pressure for another 10 minutes (no cooking).

6. Then open the vent to release more pressure (if any left)

7. Remove the valve after the floating valve in the lid drops (indicating it is safe to remove). Note: Take precautions removing the frittata pan. If you see liquid on top, it will solidify soon after some evaporation while cooling.

8. Serve the dish by slicing the frittata into 4 slices.

Nutrition Facts:

- Per serving: 92 calories
- 1 gram of Carbohydrates
- 6 grams of Protein
- 6 grams of Fat
- 2 grams of Saturated Fat
- 132 milligrams of Cholesterol
- 193 milligrams of Sodium
- 97 milligrams of Potassium
- 475 International Unit
- 1.7 milligrams of Vitamin C
- 80 milligrams of Calcium
- 0.7 milligrams of Iron

Ham & Asparagus Breakfast Roll-Ups

Ingredients:

- ½ pounds of asparagus stalks trimmed
- 2 tablespoons of olive oil
- Kosher salt
- Freshly ground black pepper
- 8 large eggs
- 3 tablespoons butter, divided
- 2 tablespoons of finely chopped chives, plus more for garnish
- 8 slices of ham
- 2 tablespoons of all-purpose flour
- 1/3 of a cup of whole milk
- 2/3 cup of freshly grated (shredded) Parmesan
- Pinch of nutmeg

How to Make:

1. Before starting, Heat oven to 400 degrees Fahrenheit.
2. Soak the asparagus with oil on a metal tray.
3. Add salt and pepper.
4. Roast for 10 minutes (until tender).
5. Meanwhile, melt 1 tablespoon of butter in medium heat in a pan.

6. Mix eggs in a bowl and pour it in the pan and slightly reduce the heat.

7. Stir with a spatula.

8. After the eggs seem cooked, add salt and pepper.

9. Fold in chives and remove from heat.

10. Place ham on a surface (plate, chopping board, etc.), and fill the hams with 2 tablespoons of scrambled eggs 2 to 3 asparagus spears.

11. Roll ham and put in a seam side down in a medium baking dish. (Repeat steps until all eggs and asparagus are used.

12. Melt butter in a saucepan in medium heat.

13. Add flour and frequently mix while it's cooking (until mixture darkens), then add milk.

14. Cook to a simmer and the mixture thickens slightly, then keep cooking for an extra minute.

15. Turn off heat and add, stir, and melt the Parmesan.

16. Add salt and nutmeg for flavoring.

17. Pour the mixture over the ham roll-ups and **BROIL IN OVEN** for 2 to 3 minutes (until it is lightly golden).

18. Serve and decorate with chives.

Nutrition Facts:

- Per serving: 53.7 calories
- 3.1 grams of total fat
- 1.4 grams of Saturated Fat
- 15.3 milligrams of Cholesterol
- 317.2 milligrams of Sodium

- 1.6 grams of Total Carbohydrate
- 0.6 grams of Dietary Fibre
- 0.4 grams of Sugars
- 5.1 grams of Protein

Bell Pepper Eggs

Ingredients:

- 1 bell pepper, sliced into ¼ inches' rings
- 6 eggs
- Kosher salt
- Freshly ground black peppers
- 2 tablespoons chopped chives
- 2 tablespoons chopped parsley

How to Make:

1. Before starting, heat a skillet in a medium heat then grease lightly with cooking spray.

2. Add 1 pepper ring into the skillet, cook one side for 2 minutes. Flip it, then crack an egg in the middle.

3. Add salt and pepper, then cook until the egg is cooked for 2 to 4 minutes.

4. Repeat with the other eggs, then garnish with chives and parsley.

Nutrition Facts:

- Per Serving: 121.5 Calories
- 7.9 grams of Total Gat
- 2.3 grams of Saturated Fat
- 1.0 grams of Polyunsaturated Fat
- 3.4 grams of Monounsaturated Fat
- 256 milligrams of Cholesterol
- 151 milligrams of Sodium

- 161.7 milligrams of Potassium
- 4 grams of Total Carbohydrate
- 1 gram of Dietary Fibre
- 0 gram of Sugar
- 8.6 grams of Protein
- Vitamin A 63.9%
- Vitamin B-12 10.4%
- Vitamin B-6 10.4%
- Vitamin C 155.8%
- Calcium 5.5%
- Copper 2.1%
- Folate 98%
- Iron 6.2%
- Manganese 3.7%
- Niacin 1.5%
- Pantothenic Acid 8.0%
- Phosphorus Acid 12.8%
- Riboflavin 19.1%
- Selenium 27.2%
- Thiamin 4.7%
- Zinc 5.1%

Everything Keto Bagels

Ingredients:

- 2 cups of Almond flour
- 1 tablespoon of baking powder
- 3 cups of shredded mozzarella cheese
- 2 ounces of cream cheese
- 2 large eggs plus 1 large egg lightly beaten
- 3 tablespoons everything bagel seasoning

How to Make:

1. Before starting, heat the oven to 400 degrees Fahrenheit.

2. Line 2 rimmed metal trays (baking sheets) with parchment paper.

3. Mix almond flour with baking powder in a large bowl.

4. Combine the mozzarella cheese and cream cheese in another medium-sized bowl (that can withstand being microwaved) and microwave for 30 seconds, then stir (repeat the microwave and stir action for a total of 8 rounds) totalling 2 minutes.

5. Scrape the mixture into the bowl with the almond flour mixture and add the two eggs, mix them until they are combined.

6. Divide the dough into 8 portions and roll each into a ball.

7. Shape each into a bagel, then place them on the metal trays.

8. Brush the top of each bagel with beaten egg and sprinkle with everything bagel seasoning.

9. Bake the bagels on the middle rack for 20 to 24 minutes (until bagel turns golden brown). Let it cool (10 minutes recommended).

Nutrition Facts:

- Per serving: 449 Calories

- 35.5 grams of Fat

- 10 grams of Carbohydrates

- 4 grams of Fibre

- 27.8 grams of Fibre

Keto Sausage Breakfast Sandwich

Ingredients:

- Cooking spray for pan
- 1 tablespoon of olive oil
- 2 large eggs
- Kosher salt
- Freshly ground black pepper
- ¼ cup of pizza sauce, divided
- ¼ cup of shredded mozzarella, divided
- 10 mini pepperoni
- Freshly grated (shredded) Parmesan
- Dried oregano

How to Make:

1. Use cooking spray on a medium skillet and the inside of a mason jar lid (glass jar), and heat skillet (pan) in medium heat.

2. Put the mason jar on the center of the skillet and crack 1 egg inside it.

3. Add half the pizza sauce, half the cheese, half the pepperoni. Cover with lid and cook until egg white is set and cheese is melted, 4 to 5 minutes. (Repeat with remaining ingredients).

4. Top with Parmesan and oregano, season with salt and pepper, and serve.

Zucchini Egg Cups

Ingredients:

- 2 zucchinis, peeled into strips
- ¼ pound of ham, chopped
- ½ cups of cherry tomatoes, quartered
- 8 eggs
- ½ cups heavy cream
- Kosher salt
- Freshly ground black pepper
- ½ tablespoon of dried oregano
- 1 cup of pinch red pepper flakes
- 1 cup of shredded cheddar
- Muffin tin
- Cooking spray

How to Make:

1. Before starting, make sure zucchinis are peeled into strips, and the hams are chopped. Heat the oven to 400 degrees Fahrenheit and spray a muffin tin with cooking spray.

2. Place the zucchini strips inside the muffin (in the form of a crust) and sprinkle ham and cherry tomatoes inside each crust.

3. Mix eggs, heavy, cream, oregano, and red pepper flakes then season with salt and pepper in a bowl and add salt and pepper.

4. Pour the mixture over the ham and tomatoes inside the zucchini strips.

5. Bake all for 30 minutes (the eggs will hint signs of being done).

Nutrition Facts:

- Per serving: 197.4 Calories
- 13.7 grams of Total Fat
- 6 grams of Saturated Fat
- 2.1 grams of Polyunsaturated Fat
- 4.2 grams of Monounsaturated Fat
- 370 milligrams of Cholesterol
- 203.1 milligrams of Sodium
- 289.4 milligrams of Potassium
- Total Carbohydrate 5.9 grams
- 2.1 grams of Dietary Fibre
- 0.8 grams of Sugars
- 13.4 grams of Protein
- Vitamin A 22.1%
- Vitamin B-12 16%
- Vitamin B-6 11.8%
- Vitamin C 6.2%
- Vitamin C 20%
- Vitamin E 0.4%
- Calcium 8.6%
- Copper 2.7%

- Folate 14.8%
- Iron 9.6%
- Magnesium 3.1%
- Manganese6.5%
- Niacin 1.2%
- Pantothenic Acid 0.8%
- Phosphorus 23.9%
- Riboflavin 21.4%
- Selenium 0.6%
- Thiamin 2.0%
- Zinc 8.9%

Keto-Friendly Cereal

Ingredients:

- Cooking spray
- 1 cup of almonds chopped
- 1 cup of walnuts, chopped
- 1 cup of unsweetened coconut flakes
- ¼ cup of sesame seeds
- 2 tablespoons flax seeds
- 2 tablespoons chia seeds
- ½ tablespoon ground clove
- ½ teaspoon ground cinnamon
- 1 teaspoon of pure vanilla extract
- 1 teaspoon of kosher salt
- 1 large white egg
- ¼ melted coconut oil

How to Make:

1. Before starting, heat the oven to 350 degrees Fahrenheit and grease a baking sheet with cooking spray.

2. Mix the almonds, walnuts, coconut flakes, sesame seeds, flax seeds, and chia seeds in a large bowl.

3. In a separate bowl, beat egg until foams are seen and add to the mixture then stir into granola.

4. Add coconut oil and stir until a single texture is formed.

5. Pour onto prepared metal tray (baking sheet) and spread into an even layer.

6. Bake for 20 to 25 minutes (or until color becomes golden).

7. Stir slowly, let it cool completely.

Nutrition Facts:

- Per serving: 90 Calories
- 3.5 grams of Total Fat
- 0 grams of Saturated Fat
- 0 grams of Trans Fat
- 0 milligrams of Cholesterol
- 90 grams of Sodium
- 20 milligrams of Potassium
- 11 grams of Total Carbohydrates
- 6 grams of Dietary Fibre
- 0 grams of Sugar
- 10 grams of Protein
- Calcium 3.9%
- Iron 6.1%

Low-Carb Breakfast Pizza

Ingredients:

- 4 large eggs
- 2 ½ shredded mozzarella
- ¼ grated Parmesan and some more for decorating (optional)
- Kosher Salt
- Freshly ground black pepper
- ¼ teaspoon dried oregano
- Pinch red pepper flakes
- 2 tablespoon pizza sauce
- ¼ mini pepperoni
- ½ chopped Green Bell Pepper

How to Make:

1. Before starting, Heat oven to 400 degrees Fahrenheit and line a metal tray (baking sheet) with parchment paper.

2. Combine eggs, 2 cups of mozzarella, and Parmesan in a bowl.

3. Stir until combined, then add season with salt, pepper, oregano, and red pepper flakes.

4. Spread mixture into a ½ inch thick round on a baking sheet

5. Bake to 12 minutes (until lightly golden).

6. Spread pizza sauce on top of baked crust. Topping with remaining mozzarella, pepperoni, and bell pepper.

7. Bake pizza for about 10 minutes (until sighting signs of melting cheese and crust is crispy),

8. Crust is crispy, about 10 minutes more. Option to add Parmesan sprinkled on top and finally serve.

Nutrition Facts:

- Per Serving: 300 Calories (4 slices)
- 25 grams of Total Fat
- 622 milligrams of Sodium
- 6 grams of Total Carbohydrates
- 27 grams of Protein

Jalapeño Popper Egg Cups

Ingredients:

- 12 slices of bacon
- 10 large eggs
- ¼ cup of sour cream
- ½ cup of shredded Cheddar
- ½ cup of shredded mozzarella
- 2 jalapeños, 1 minced and 1 thin slice
- 1 teaspoon of garlic powder
- Kosher salt
- Freshly ground black pepper
- Cooking Spray (for nonstick skillet)

How to Make:

1. Before starting, Heat oven at 375 degrees Fahrenheit.

2. Cook bacon in a skillet at medium heat (until color changes to a little brown).

3. Use a paper towel to drain the bacon of oil.

4. Whisk eggs, sour cream, cheeses, minced jalapeño, and garlic powder in a large bowl.

5. Season with salt and pepper.

6. Spray muffin tin with cooking spray and line each bacon on each tin cup.

7. Pour the mixture into each tin cup (2/3 fills) and add jalapeño slice at the top for each.

8. Bake for 20 minutes (until the eggs don't look wet anymore). Cool slightly before removing from the muffin tin. Serve.

Nutrition Facts:

- Per serving: 157 Calories
- 12 grams of Total Fat
- 1 gram of Total Carbs
- 9 grams of Protein

Spaghetti squash Bolognese

Ingredients:

- 1 large spaghetti squash
- 3 tablespoon thrive algae oil
- 1 and ¼ teaspoons of sea salt (1 is for taste)
- ½ chopped medium yellow onion
- 5 minced cloves garlic
- 1 tablespoon of dried oregano
- 1 tablespoon of dried parsley
- 2 teaspoons of dried thyme
- 2 teaspoons of dried rosemary
- 2 teaspoons of dried basil
- ¼ teaspoon of cayenne
- 1 pound of grass-fed ground beef
- 28 ounces of can crushed tomatoes
- 3 tablespoons of tomato paste
- 2 teaspoons of pure maple syrup (optional)

How to Make:

1. Before Starting, Heat the oven to 415 degrees Fahrenheit.

2. Cut the tip and tail off the spaghetti squash and use a spoon to scoop out the seeds.

3. Drizzle the flesh with 1 tablespoon of algae oil and sprinkle with ¼ teaspoon of sea salt.

4. Place squash on a baking sheet cut-side down and roast for 45 to 50 minutes, or until very tender.

5. Meanwhile, use a large skillet in medium heat to cook 2 tablespoons of algae oil.

6. Add onion and cook & stir for about 8 minutes (until onion is translucent).

7. Add garlic and herbs (oregano through cayenne) and continue cooking for 3 minutes.

8. Add the sea salt, crushed tomatoes, tomato paste, and pure maple syrup.

9. Make way for the ground beef in the pan.

10. Cook the beef for 3 minutes on both sides (until its brown).

11. Use a spatula to mix the meat with what in the pan.

12. Add 1 teaspoon of sea salt, crushed tomatoes, tomato paste, and maple syrup. Don't cook the meat all the way through just yet.

13. Stir & cook for 30 minutes to an hour, depending on when the sauce starts to make bubbles.

14. Depending on the taste, add more sea salt.

15. Pour on top of spaghetti squash with fresh basil.

Nutrition Facts:

- Per Serving: 300 Calories

- 12 grams of Total Fat

- 2 grams of Saturated Fat

- 0 grams of Trans Fat

- 0 grams of Cholesterol
- 1.82 grams of Sodium
- 40 grams Total Carbohydrates
- 9 grams of Dietary Fibre
- 13 grams of Sugars
- 8 grams of Protein

Spring rolls with lime-peanut sauce

Ingredients:

- ½ cup of unsalted creamy peanut butter
- ¼ cup and 1 tablespoon of warm water
- 2 tablespoons freshly squeezed lime juice
- 1 tablespoon + 1 teaspoon soy sauce.
- 1 tablespoon rice vinegar
- 2 teaspoons of grated fresh ginger root
- 1 teaspoon of sriracha sauce
- 2 ounces of dried brown rice noodles
- 8 round brown rice paper wrappers (plus extra for any mistakes!!)
- 1 pound of cooked shrimp (deveined and peeled)
- 1.5 cups of thinly sliced red cabbage
- 1 sizeable sliced orange/yellow/red bell pepper into thin strips
- 1 pitted and sliced ripe avocado
- Baby, red lettuce leaves
- Fresh cilantro leaves
- Fresh mint leaves

How to Make:

- Combine all of the ingredients in the bowl of a small food processor (mixer, blender), then start blending until the solution is smooth (if the solution is too thick, experiment by adding a teaspoon of water and blend/mix/pulse again).

- Add salt and pepper to mix.

- Boil water in a large pot and cook the brown rice noodles (according to the package instructions).

- Drain any excess water by letting it cool.

- Fill a large bowl with hot water.

- Working with one paper at a time.

- Soak the brown rice paper in hot water for 15 seconds

- Lay 3 to 4 six shrimps halves in a row, cut side up in the center of the rice paper, leaving 1 to 1.5 inches on either side of the shrimp.

- Put the cooked rice noodles on top of the shrimp.

- Add toppings of shredded red cabbage, 2 to 3 strips of bell pepper, two slices of avocado and baby lettuce leaf, and fresh cilantro (in that order).

- Fold over the bottom half of the wrapper (brown rice paper) over the filling, holding it in place.

- Roll it tightly yet carefully not to rip the paper apart from top to bottom. (Repeat for the remaining).

- Serve with creamy peanut butter as a dipping sauce.

Nutrition Facts:

- Per Serving: 170 Calories

- 9 grams of Total Fat

- 1.5 grams of Saturated Fat

- 0 grams of Trans Fat

- 20 milligrams of Cholesterol

- 440 milligrams of Sodium

- 18 grams of Total Carbohydrates

- 2 grams of Dietary Fibre
- 1 gram of Sugars
- 4 grams of Protein
- Vitamin A 30%
- Vitamin C 8%
- Calcium 2%
- Iron 4%

Grilled Taco Chickens

Ingredients:

- 1 pound of Boneless skinless chicken breasts/thighs
- 2 tablespoons of taco seasoning
- 3 cloves of minced garlic
- 3 tablespoons of olive oil
- 8 rinsed leaves of Romaine Lettuce
- 1 dried avocado
- 1 dried tomato
- ¼ cup onion diced
- ½ cup loosely packed cilantro
- ½ cup of Greek Yogurt/sour cream/mayonnaise
- 1 jalapeño (optional)
- ½ lime juice
- Pinch of salt

How to Make:

1. In a large bowl/zip-seal bag, add the chicken, 2 cloves of garlic, 1 tablespoon of olive oil and spice, and taco seasoning.

2. Refrigerate for 15 to 30 minutes (can go up to 24 hours).

3. Take out the chicken (only) and heat it on a pan for 9 to 10 minutes on each side at medium-high heat.

4. Place the romaine lettuce, avocado, tomato, and onion (leave some of the items mentioned for gar-

nishing) in a food processor (blender, mixer, etc.) for 1 minute (until it is creamy).

5. Layer lettuce wraps with chicken and the left-over ingredients not put in the blender. Drizzle with the blended mixture. Now it's ready to be served.

Nutrition Facts:

- Per Serving: 185 Calories
- 6.2 grams of Total Fat
- 2.5 grams of Saturated Fat
- 0.1 gram of Trans Fat
- 1.6 grams of Polyunsaturated Fat
- 1.6 grams of Monounsaturated Fat
- 28 milligrams of Cholesterol
- 601 milligrams of Sodium
- 213 milligrams of Potassium
- 19 grams of Total Carbohydrates
- 1.2 grams of Dietary Fibre
- 1.3 grams of Sugars
- 13 grams of Protein
- Vitamin A 3.9%
- Vitamin C 0.3%
- Calcium 9.2%
- Iron 8.7 %

Zucchini and beet 'noodle' salad

Ingredients:

- 2 tablespoons of extra virgin olive oil
- 3 minced garlic cloves
- 16 ounces of zucchini squash
- 1 small beet
- ½ teaspoon soy sauce
- ½ teaspoon salt
- 1/8 teaspoon of ground black pepper
- 2 tablespoons of freshly squeezed lime juice
- 1 teaspoon of sesame oil
- 3 tablespoons of chopped cilantro leaves

How to Make:

1. Before starting, heat pan/skillet over high heat.

2. Add the extra virgin olive oil and cook for 15 seconds.

3. Turn off heat and add garlic and sesame seeds to the skillet/pan.

4. Let it cool to room temperature.

5. Meanwhile, trim the ends of the zucchini squash and beet.

6. Use a vegetable spiralizer (vegetable slicing machine).

7. Place the zucchini noodles and beet noodles in **separate** bowls.

8. Add the cooled garlic oil into the zucchini noodles and gently toss until the oil is evenly coated on the noodles.

9. Refrigerate both bowls of noodles.

10. After cooling, whisk together all the dressing ingredients except cilantro leaves.

11. Gently toss together with the zucchini noodles (both) and cilantro leaves. Ready to Serve.

Nutrition Facts:

- Per Serving: 280 Calories
- 16 grams of Total Fat
- 3.5 grams of Saturated Fat
- 0 grams of Trans Fat
- 0 milligrams of Cholesterol
- 110 milligrams of Sodium
- 1031 milligrams of Potassium
- 25 grams of Total Carbohydrates
- 6 grams of Dietary Fibre
- 10 grams of Sugars
- 11 grams of Protein
- Calcium 19%
- Iron 28%

Stuffed Portobello Pizzas

Ingredients:

- 6 Portobello mushroom caps stems removed, washed and dried with a paper towel

- 2 tablespoons extra-virgin olive oil

- 2 teaspoons minced garlic

- 6 teaspoons Italian seasoning/oregano and basil leaf blend/

- ¾ cups of pizza sauce (garlic and herb)

- ½ cups reduced-fat shredded mozzarella cheese/pizza cheese blend

- 30 miniature-sized pepperonis

- 6 slice thinly cherries/grape tomatoes

- Salt and pepper

How to Make:

- Before starting, **broil/grill** oven on high heat and arrange the oven shelf to the middle position.

- Mix the oil, garlic, and seasoning in a small bowl.

- Brush each mushroom's bottom with the mixture made and place them on a lightly greased metal tray.

- Fill each mushroom with 2 tablespoons of the pizza sauce per cap, ¼ cup of mozzarella cheese, 6 pepperoni miniatures, and tomato slices.

- **Broil/grill** until the cheese has melted and is golden in color.

- Serve and sprinkle with remaining Italian seasoning/oregano and basil leaf blend.

Nutrition Facts:

- Per serving: 215 Calories
- 13 grams of Total Fat
- 6.5 grams of Saturated Fat
- 0.4 gram of Trans Fat
- 1.1 grams of Polyunsaturated Fat
- 4.3 grams of Monounsaturated Fat
- 36 milligrams of Cholesterol
- 603 milligrams of Sodium
- 502 milligrams of Potassium
- 11 grams of Total Carbohydrates
- 1.9 grams of Dietary Fibre
- 4.7 grams of Sugars
- 14 grams of Protein
- Vitamin A 12%
- Vitamin C 2.7%
- Calcium 25%
- Iron 5%

Avocado sushi rolls

Ingredients:

- 80 grams of uncooked sushi rice
- 1 to 2 tablespoons of rice vinegar
- ½ tablespoons sugar
- 1 sheet seaweed nori paper
- ½ large avocado, de-seeded and cut into strips
- ½ yellow pepper, de-seeded and cut into strips
- 1 to 2 sliced leaves Iceberg lettuce
- 1 large avocado

How to Make:

1. Cook sushi rice according to the package instruction.

2. Place the sushi rice in a bowl along with sugar, rice vinegar, and let it cool.

3. Cut the seaweed paper in half and set aside.

4. Place a layer of cling film on a bamboo mat to prevent the rice from sticking.

5. Place the seaweed paper on top of the bamboo mat, use a wet spoon, and add half of the sushi rice and spread evenly on the seaweed paper.

6. Flip the rice along with the seaweed paper.

7. Put vegetables (sliced) on top of the seaweed paper.

8. Roll and gently press the sushi into square shapes. (Repeat until all is used).

9. Chop 1 full large avocado in half, and scrape all of its insides.

10. The other avocado (0.5) should be sliced, carefully while keeping its full shape and then those slices are to be moved to the top of the sushi roll, and cover them with the cling film to press the avocado slices onto the rolls with the others.

11. Slice each roll into 8 pieces of sushi.

12. Remove the cling film, and it's ready to serve with soy sauce and wasabi.

Nutrition Facts:

- Per Serving: 321 Calories
- 11 grams of Total Fat
- 1.6 grams of Saturated Fat
- 1.4 grams of Polyunsaturated Fat
- 6.8 grams of Monounsaturated Fat
- 0 milligrams of Cholesterol
- 34 milligrams of Sodium
- 422 milligrams of Potassium
- 51 grams of Total Carbohydrates
- 4.7 grams of Dietary Fibre
- 0.3 gram of Sugars
- 6.5 grams of Protein
- Vitamin A 2.3%
- Vitamin C 10%
- Calcium 1.1%
- Iron 8.4%

Rainbow salad bowl

Ingredients:

- 1 handful of fresh spinach
- 1 handful of od de-stemmed and chopped red cabbage
- 1 small raw shredded carrot
- 1 peeled, chopped and roasted acorn squash
- 1 steamed chopped broccoli
- 1 tablespoon sunflower seeds
- 1 tablespoon of pumpkin seeds
- ¼ of a diced avocado
- 1 Dried kelp flakes
- ¼ tablespoon of water
- 1 big chunk of peeled fresh ginger
- 3 tablespoons of tahini
- 2 tablespoons of pure maple syrup
- 2 tablespoons of apple cider vinegar
- 1 tablespoon of soy sauce/gluten-free tamari

How to Make:

1. Blend the spinach, kale, beet, red cabbage, carrot, acorn squash, broccoli, seeds, avocado, and kelp flakes in a food processor (blender, mixer, etc.).

2. Either mix in a bowl or separately add the water, ginger, tahini, maple syrup, miso paste, apple cider vinegar, soy sauce/gluten-free tamari to the mixture. Bona Petite.

Cashew-topped pumpkin soup

Ingredients:

- 1 tablespoon of oil/butter
- ½ chopped onion
- 1 teaspoon of kosher salt
- 2 cloves of peeled and minced garlic
- 4 cups of chicken/vegetable broth
- 15 ounces of can pure vegetable broth
- ¼ teaspoon of ground turmeric
- ½ cup of roasted salted cashews plus extra for garnishing
- ¼ cup of roasted salted pepitas for garnish
- 1 dried parsley for garnishing (optional)

How to Make:

1. Cook onions in oil and butter in the pot over medium high until it is translucent.

2. Add salt pepper and minced garlic—Cook for 1 to 2 minutes.

3. Now heat at medium low, add chicken/vegetable and pumpkin to the pot and stir.

4. Add turmeric, basil, and cumin. Simmer and stir.

5. Add 2 cups of the soup and ½ cup of cashews to a blender for 30 to 45 seconds (until it is creamy). Note: Take precautions using the blender. It is optional to add the mixture back to the pot with onion pieces for texture.

6. Depending on the taste, add as much kosher salt and pepper as needed.

7. Now could be served in a bowl(s) (depending on how much soup it is left) and garnished with pepitas, chopped cashews, and parsley.

Cauliflower fried rice

Ingredients:

- 1 24 ounces of rinsed cauliflower
- 1 tablespoon of sesame oil
- 2 egg white
- 1 large egg
- Pinch of salt
- Cooking spray
- ½ small diced onion
- ½ cup of frozen peas and carrots
- 2 minced garlic cloves
- 5 diced white scallions
- 5 diced green scallions
- 3 tablespoons of soy sauce (optional: add more for taste)
- Cooking Spray

How to Make:

1. Let the cauliflower dry.

2. Chop and place half of the cauliflower into a food processor (blender, mixer) until it has a texture that of rice. (Repeat for the remaining cauliflower.)

3. Mix egg, egg white with salt in a bowl.

4. Heat a large pan at medium heat then spray with cooking oil.

5. Add the egg mixture into the pan. Make sure all sides are cooked well.

6. Add the sesame oil and cook the onions and scallion whites, the **frozen** peas and carrots for 3 to 4 minutes at medium high.

7. Add the cauliflower, soy sauce, rice to the pan.

8. Mix well, then cover and cook for 5 to 6 minutes, occasionally stirring the mixture.

9. When the cauliflower is a little crispy, add the egg, then turn off the heat and mix in scallion greens. Now it's ready to be served.

Nutrition Facts:

- Per serving: 321 Calories

- 11 grams of total fat

- 1.6 grams of saturated fat

- 1.4 grams of polyunsaturated fat

- 6.8 grams of monounsaturated fat

- 0 milligram of cholesterol

- 34 milligrams of Sodium

- 422 milligrams of potassium

- 51 grams of total carbohydrates

- 4.7 grams of dietary fibre

- 0.3 grams of Sugars

- 6.5 grams of protein

- Vitamin A 2.3

- Vitamin C 10

- Calcium 1.1

- Iron 8.4

Almond-citrus salad

Ingredients:

- 1/3 cup of orange juice
- 2 tablespoons of white wine vinegar
- 2 tablespoons of vegetable oil
- 1 tablespoon of honey
- 2 teaspoons of grated fresh ginger
- ¼ teaspoon of salt
- 1/8 teaspoon of red pepper flakes
- 2 peeled and segmented grapefruits
- 2 peeled and segmented navel oranges
- ¼ cup of chopped red onion
- 6 cups of lightly packed torn into a bite-sized pieces' spinach leaves
- 2/3 cups of toasted slivered almonds

How to Make:

1. Apply juice, vinegar, oil, honey, ginger, salt, and pepper flakes into a blender and blend.

2. Combine fruit, onion, and dressing and leave the mix in a bowl for 10 minutes (up to an hour).

3. Prepare four plates with spinach and add a fruit mixture over on each spinach

4. Place almonds (proportions are based on your liking) on baking pan at 350 degrees Fahrenheit' oven and bake for 5 to 10 minutes (until almonds are light brown.

5. Sprinkle the almonds over the meal. Now you are ready to serve.

Nutrition Facts

- Per serving: 170 Calories
- 14 grams of Total Fat
- 0 grams of Trans Fat
- 0 milligrams of Cholesterol
- 280 milligrams of Sodium
- 7 grams of Total Carbohydrates
- 3 grams of Dietary Fibre
- 2 grams of Sugars
- 6 grams of Protein
- Vitamin A 0%
- Vitamin C 0%
- Calcium 8%
- Iron 6%

Mini spinach-tomato quiche

Ingredients:

- 1 tablespoon of olive oil
- 2 cups of trimmed and washed fresh spinach leaves
- 4 large eggs
- 2/3 cup heavy cream/milk/half of each
- 1/3 cup crumbled feta cheese
- 1-2 diced plum tomatoes
- 2 cloves of minced garlic
- Salt and freshly ground black pepper
- 1 cup all-purpose flour
- ½ teaspoon salt
- ¼ cup of olive oil
- ¼ cup of ice-cold water
- 9 to 10 inches' Pie dish

How to Make:

1. Mix the flour and salt in a medium bowl.

2. In another bowl, beat mix oil and water until it thickens.

3. Pour the flour salt mix into the other bowl and mix again.

4. Place dough into the pie dish and make sure you thin out the dough.

5. Set the oven to 350 degrees Fahrenheit, **then after it is heated,** make the quiche filling.

6. Spread the feta cheese onto the bottom of the crust.

7. Toss in the spinach and cook until wilted; after that, spread the spinach over the cheese.

8. Mix the eggs, garlic, heavy cream/milk, and season with salt and pepper in a separate bowl.

9. Pour this mixture over the feta cheese and spinach.

10. Add toppings of tomatoes.

11. **Optional** to add other toppings like ground pepper and extra feta cheese. (Optional to skip this step.)

12. Fill with quiche mixture and bake at 350 degrees Fahrenheit for 35 to 45 minutes until fully baked and set. Now it's ready to serve.

Nutrition Facts:

- Per Serving: 460 Calories
- 34 grams of Total Fat
- 19 grams of Saturated Fat
- 0 grams of Trans Fat
- 245 milligrams of Cholesterol
- 530 milligrams of Sodium
- 25 grams of Total Carbohydrates
- 1 gram of Dietary Fibre
- 4 grams of Sugars
- 15 grams of Protein
- Vitamin a 45%
- Vitamin C 15%
- Calcium 30%

- Iron 15%

Creamy mushroom soup

Ingredients:

- 4 tablespoons of butter
- 1 tablespoon of oil
- 2 diced onions
- 4 cloves of minced garlic
- ½ pounds of fresh brown sliced mushrooms
- 4 teaspoons of chopped, divided thyme
- ½ cup Marsala red/white wine
- 6 tablespoons of all-purpose flour
- 4 cups of low-sodium chicken broth or stock
- 1 to 2 teaspoons of black cracked pepper
- 2 beef bouillon crumbled cubes
- 1 cup of heavy cream/half milk half evaporated milk
- Chopped fresh parsley and thyme to serve

How to Make:

1. Set a large pot to medium-high and cook butter and oil until it melts.

2. Add onions and cook for 2 to 3 minutes.

3. Sprinkle flour over mushrooms and mix well and cook for 2 minutes.

4. Set heat to low-medium heat and add salt, pepper, and crumbled bouillon cubes.

5. Cover the pot and let it simmer for 10 to 15 minutes. Stir from time to time.

6. Set heat to low, then add the heavy cream/half-cream half milk into the pan and cook until it's the solution is thick.

7. Mix in parsley and remaining thyme. Now it is ready to be served.

Nutrition Facts:

- Per Serving: 405 Calories
- 34 grams of Total Fat
- 20 grams of Saturated Fat
- 1.2 grams of Tran Fat
- 1.7 grams of Polyunsaturated Fat
- 9.8 grams of Monounsaturated Fat
- 92 milligrams of Cholesterol
- 173 milligrams of Sodium
- 476 milligrams of Potassium
- 16 grams of Total Carbohydrates
- 2.4 grams of Dietary Fibre
- 6.6 grams of Sugar
- 5.3 grams of Protein
- Vitamin A 67%
- Vitamin C 19%
- Calcium 8.2%
- Iron 8.4%

Shirataki noodle soup

Ingredients:

- 2 packs of shirataki noodles
- 1.5 pounds of chicken drumstick
- 2 cups of chicken stock
- 2 cups of water
- 3 tablespoons of olive oil
- 2 stalks of chopped celery
- ½ of chopped onion
- 2 cloves of chopped garlic
- 3 tablespoons of coconut amino
- ½ teaspoon of smoked paprika
- 1 teaspoon of black pepper
- 1 teaspoon of thyme
- 1 teaspoon of bouillon powder
- ½ teaspoon cayenne pepper (optional)
- Salt
- Parsley and other herbs for garnishing (optional)

How to Make:

1. Wash chicken and leave to dry
2. Add oil to instant pot and press the cook button.
3. Add celery and stir for a few more minutes till it just begins to soften.

4. Add the chicken, water, chicken stock, smoked paprika pepper, black pepper, thyme, bouillon powder, cayenne pepper, and salt into the pot.

5. Switch the instant pot to manual mode and cook on high pressure for 20 minutes.

6. Take out the chicken, shred to pieces and put the pieces back in the pot.

7. Add the coconut amino and salt.

8. **Optional** to freeze the noodles before adding them.

9. Switch instant pot to sauté mode and add the shirataki noodles.

10. Simmer for 5 minutes.

11. Garnish with parsley with a personal decorative touch. Now it's ready to be served.

Nutrition Facts:

- Per Serving: 85 Calories
- 4 grams of Total Fat
- 0.5 grams of Saturated Fat
- 0 grams of Trans Fat
- 0 milligrams of Cholesterol
- 305 milligrams of Sodium
- 11 grams of Total Carbohydrates
- 5 grams of Dietary Fibre
- 2 grams of Sugars
- 1 gram of Protein
- Vitamin A 0%

- Vitamin C 3%
- Calcium 4%
- Iron 2%

BLT Chicken Salad

- ½ cup of mayonnaise
- 3 to 4 tablespoons of barbecue sauce
- 2 tablespoons of chopped onion
- 1 tablespoon of lemon juice
- ¼ teaspoon of pepper
- 8 cups of torn salad greens
- 2 chopped large tomatoes
- ½ pounds of cooked and cubed boneless skinless chicken breasts
- 10 cooked and crumbled bacon strips
- 2 sliced hard-boiled large eggs

How to Make:

1. Prepare a bowl, then add and mix mayonnaise, barbecue, onion, lemon juice, and pepper. Cover the bowl and put it in the refrigerator (until it is at a cool temperature). This will be the dressing.

2. Prepare another bowl and add the salads, then the tomatoes, chicken, bacon, and eggs.

3. Add the contents of the dressing ball to the large bowl.

Nutrition Facts:

- Per serving: 281 Calories
- 19 grams of Fat
- 4 grams of Saturated Fat

- 112 milligrams of Cholesterol
- 324 milligrams of Sodium
- 5 grams of Carbohydrates
- 23 grams of Protein

Zesty Steak Chili

Ingredients:

- 4 pounds of 1-inch cubes (cut) beef top round steak
- 4 minced garlic cloves
- ¼ cup of canola oil
- 3 cups of chopped onion
- 2 (¾) cups of water
- 2 cups of sliced celery
- 3 cans (14 to ½ ounces each) of diced undrained tomatoes
- 2 cans (15 ounces each) of tomato sauce (no salt)
- 1 jar (16 ounces) of salsa
- 3 tablespoons of chili powder
- 2 teaspoons of ground cumin
- 1 teaspoon of salt (optional)
- 1 teaspoon of pepper
- ¼ cup of all-purpose flour
- ¼ cup of yellow cornmeal
- Shredded reduced-fat cheddar cheese (optional, for garnish)
- Reduced-fat sour cream (optional, for garnish)
- Sliced green onions (optional, for garnish)
- Sliced ripe olives (optional, for garnish)

How to Make:

- Prepare a Dutch oven with canola oil. Cook steak and garlic until the color turns brown.

- Add onion to the Dutch oven and cook for 5 minutes.

- Add water and the 2 cups (3/4) of water and stir (until the solutions combine).

- Add the celery, diced tomatoes, no-salt tomato sauce, salsa, chili powder, ground cumin, salt (optional) and pepper, then boil.

- After boiling, reduce the heat (no longer boiling) and make it simmer for 2 hours.

- Add the flour, cook and stir for 2 minutes.

- Once it thickens, pour a serving and garnish with optional ingredients.

Nutrition Facts:

- Per Serving: 200 Calories (1 cup)

- 6 grams of Fat

- 51 milligrams of Cholesterol

- 247 milligrams of Sodium

- 13 grams of Total Carbohydrates

- 3 grams of Fibre

- 7 grams of Sugars

- 22 grams of Protein

Slow-Cooker Chicken Taco Salad

Ingredients:

- 3 teaspoons of chili powder
- 1 teaspoon of seasoned salt
- 1 teaspoon of pepper
- ½ teaspoon of ground chipotle
- ½ teaspoon of pepper
- ½ teaspoon of paprika
- ¼ teaspoon of dried oregano
- ¼ teaspoon of crushed red pepper flakes
- ½ pounds of boneless skinless chicken breast
- 1 cup of chicken broth
- 9 cups of torn romaine
- Sliced avocado (optional, toppings)
- Shredded cheddar cheese (optional, toppings)
- Chopped Tomato (optional, toppings)
- Sliced green onions (optional, toppings)
- Ranch Salad dressing (optional, toppings)
- Slow Cooker

How to Make:

- Prepare a bowl and add **all** the seasonings and mix them.
- Get the chicken and soak it with the seasonings.

- Place the chicken in the slow cooker too and add the chicken broth.

- Cook while cover for 3 to 4 hours.

- Take out the chicken and let it cool.

- Prepare a plate with the romaine and place the chicken over.

- (Optional) Add toppings. The meal is ready.

Nutrition Facts:

- Per Serving: 143 Calories (3/4 cups)

- 3 grams of Total Fat

- 1 gram of Saturated Fat

- 63 milligrams of Cholesterol

- 516 grams of Sodium

- 4 grams of Total Carbohydrates

- 2 grams of Fibre

- 1 gram of Sugars

- 24 grams of Protein

Ham Salad

Ingredients:

- ¾ cup mayonnaise
- ½ cup chopped celery
- ¼ cup sliced green onions
- 2 tablespoons minced fresh chives
- 1 tablespoon honey
- 2 teaspoons of spicy brown mustard
- ½ teaspoon of Worcestershire sauce
- ½ teaspoon of seasoned salt
- 5 cups of diced fully cooked ham/turkey
- 1/3 cup of chopped pecans and almonds, toasted
- Split slider buns (optional)

How to Make:

1. Prepare a bowl with the ingredients mention here: mayonnaise, celery onions, chives, honey, brown mustard, Worcestershire sauce, and seasoned salt. Mix them.

2. Rub the ingredients on the ham/turkey then place the turkey in the refrigerator.

3. Once it's cooled, and the pecans and almonds.

4. (Optional) Add the buns. The meal is now ready.

Nutrition Facts:

- Per serving: 254 Calories (1/2 cup ham salad)
- 20 grams of Total Fat

- 3 grams of Saturated Fat
- 43 milligrams of Cholesterol
- 1023 milligrams of Sodium
- 4 grams of Total Carbohydrates
- 1 gram of Fibre
- 2 grams of Sugars
- 16 grams of Protein

Tomato-Melon Chicken Salad

Ingredients:

- 4 (cut into wedges) tomatoes
- 2 cups of cubed seedless watermelon
- 1 cup of fresh raspberries
- ¼ cup of minced fresh basil
- ¼ cup of olive oil
- 2 tablespoons of balsamic vinegar
- ¼ teaspoon of salt
- ¼ teaspoon of pepper
- 9 cups of torn mixed salad greens
- 4 (4 ounces each) sliced grilled chicken breasts

How to Make:

- Prepare a large bowl with tomatoes, watermelon, and raspberries. Mix them.
- Prepare a small bowl with the whisked mixture of basil, oil, vinegar, salt, and pepper.
- Use the mixture in the small ball to drizzle over the contents of the more giant bowl.

- Divide the salad greens among 6 serving plates (or 1/6 if it's just one person).
- Add the contents of the large bowl as toppings with the chicken over the plate. Ready to serve.

Nutrition Facts:

- Per serving: 266 calories

- 13 grams of Total Fat
- 2 grams of Saturated Fat
- 64 milligrams of Cholesterol
- 215 milligrams of Sodium
- 15 grams of Total Carbohydrates
- 4 grams of Fibre
- 9 grams of Sugars
- 26 grams of Protein

Focaccia Sandwiches

Ingredients:

- 1/3 cup of mayonnaise
- 1 can (4 and 1/4 ounces) of drained, chopped ripe olives
- 1 split focaccia bread (about 12 ounces)
- 4 romaine leaves
- ¼ pound shaves deli ham
- 1 (sliced into rings) medium sweet red pepper
- ¼ pound cut deli turkey

- 1 large tomato, thinly sliced
- ¼ pound of thinly sliced salami
- 1 jar (7 ounces) of drained roasted sweet red peppers
- 4 to 6 slices of provolone cheese

How to Make:

- Prepare a small bowl with mayonnaise and olives.
- Use that as to spread over the **bottom half** of the bread.
- Layer the rest of the ingredients and then place top bread.
- Cut into 24 wedges.

Nutrition Facts:

- Per serving: 113 calories
- 6 grams of fat

- 2 grams of Saturated Fat
- 13 milligrams of Cholesterol
- 405 milligrams of Sodium
- 9 grams of Total Carbohydrates
- 1 gram of Sugars
- 1 gram of Fibre
- 5 grams of Protein

RECIPES FOR DINNER

Grilled Beef-Mushroom Burgers

Ingredients:

- 4 ounces of sliced button mushrooms
- 1 pound of 90% lean ground sirloin
- 2 tablespoons olive oil
- 1/8 teaspoon of black pepper
- ¾ of teaspoons of divided kosher salt
- Divided 1/3 cup of chopped cucumber
- ¼ cup of plain whole milk/Greek yogurt
- 2 tablespoons of minced roasted garlic (about 4 large cloves).
- 1 tablespoon of fresh lemon juice
- 1 tablespoon of chopped fresh flat-leaf parsley
- 8 large butter lettuce leaves
- 4 heirloom tomato slices
- 4 red onion slices

How to Make:

1. Before starting, heat grill/grill pan to medium high at 450 degrees Fahrenheit.

2. Place the mushrooms in a food processor (blender, mixer, vegetable splicer and such), and process until minced for 1 minute.

3. Mix mushrooms and ground sirloin, oil, pepper, and 3/8 teaspoon salt in a medium bowl; gently shape into 4 patties (4 inches) and put on a metal tray with parchment paper (baking paper, so it doesn't stick).

4. Mix the cucumber, garlic yogurt, parsley, lemon juice, and remaining 3/8 teaspoon salt in a small bowl.

5. Arrange plates for each pair of lettuce leaves (4 plates). Add toppings of each with a burger patty, tomato slice, red onion slice, and 1 tablespoon of the mixture in the small bowl. Ready to be served.

Nutrition Facts

- Per serving: 304 Calories
- 19 grams of Total Fat
- 6 grams of Saturated Fat
- 11 grams of Unsaturated Fat
- 26 grams of Protein
- 7 grams of Carbohydrate
- 1 gram of Fibre
- 3 grams of Sugars
- 0 grams of added sugars
- 447 milligrams of Sodium
- Calcium 6%
- Potassium 20%

Cauliflower Risotto with Mush-

rooms

Ingredients:

- 5 tablespoons olive oil
- 10 ounces of sliced fresh cremini mushrooms
- 6 ounces of chopped onion
- 2 teaspoons of fresh thyme leaves
- 2 teaspoons of chopped garlic
- ¼ cup of dry white wine
- 24 ounces of fresh riced cauliflower
- 1 cup of water
- ½ cup of unsalted vegetable stock
- ½ teaspoon of kosher salt
- ¼ teaspoon of black pepper
- 2 ounces of shredded and divided Parmesan cheese

How to Make:

1. Heat ½ of the olive oil on a large pan set to medium-high.

2. Add half of the mushrooms. Stir while cooking for 5 minutes (until mushrooms show a color change: brown).

3. Take out mushrooms from pan and place on a plate. (Repeat steps of olive oil and mushroom cooking with the remaining ingredients).

4. Set heat to medium, then add onion, thyme, garlic and remaining oil (2 tablespoons recommended)— Cook for 5 minutes with stirring.

5. Add wine and continue to stir and cook for 90 seconds.

6. Add cauliflower, water, and stock into the pan. Stir again.

7. Cook while covering the pan. From time to time, stir. It shall last about 10 to 12 minutes

8. Turn off heat, then mixture from the pan to the blender, and blend for 15 seconds.

9. Take out the mixture from the blender and pour it back to the pan and heat at medium.

10. Add cauliflower puree, mushrooms, salt, pepper, and ¼ cup of the cheese.

11. Cook and stir until cheese melts with the texture of cream (will take about 1 minute).

12. Sprinkle evenly with remaining ½ cup cheese and garnish with thyme leaves and serve.

Nutrition Facts:

- Per serving: 245 Calories
- 19 grams of Fat
- 60 milligrams of Cholesterol
- 7 grams of Carbohydrates
- 2 grams of Dietary Fibre

Eggs in Purgatory

Ingredients:

- ¼ cup of olive oil (save more for drizzling)
- 5 smashed garlic cloves
- Freshly ground pepper
- Kosher salt
- ½ teaspoon of crushed red pepper flakes
- 20 ounces of cherry tomatoes
- 1 bunch of Swiss chard (rainbow recommended)
- 6 large errs
- 4 thin slices of bread
- 1 lemon
- Flaky sea salt or kosher salt
- A handful of basil leaves

How to Make:

1. Heat olive oil in a medium pan/skillet at medium-high.

2. When oil simmers, add garlic and season generously with kosher salt and black pepper.

3. Cook and stir until garlic is just turning golden around the edges, for 2 minutes.

4. Stir in red pepper flakes, then add tomatoes and cook while flipping them around. (until tomatoes look plumped) and some of the skins start to split about 2 minutes.

5. Set heat to medium. Cook while covering the pan. Stir every two minutes to prevent them from sticking. Do this for 5 minutes.

6. Afterward/Meanwhile (depending on if you can multitask while stirring every 2 minutes) strip leaves off Swiss chard stems and tear into preferred sizes into a medium bowl.

7. Set heat to medium-low **after tomato mixture shows a bubbling effect**, crack an egg in different areas of the tomato sauce like states in a country (each with its area).

8. Add salt and pepper to the eggs, then cover and cook for 4 to 6 minutes.

9. Toast bread until it's crispy.

10. Drizzle bread with oil and rub bread with lemon (not peeled), and sprinkle sea salt on bread.

11. Pour lemon juice over greens and add basil, oil, kosher salt, and black pepper and mix them.

12. Take out each egg in the pan carefully (while keeping the egg intact) and put in a bowl, then season with sauce and sea salt. Now it can be garnished with salad and toasts on the sides.

Nutrition Facts:

- Per serving: 197 Calories

- 11.6 grams of Total Fat

- 3 grams of Saturated Fat

- 6 grams of Monounsaturated Fat

- 1.4 grams of Polyunsaturated Fat

- 112 milligrams of Total Omega-3 fatty acids

- 1233 milligrams of Total Omega-6 fatty acids

- 215 milligrams of Cholesterol
- 431 milligrams of Sodium
- 14. Grams of Total Carbohydrate
- 3.4 grams of Dietary Fibre
- 4.3 grams of Sugars
- 10.5 grams of Protein
- Vitamin A 11%
- Vitamin C 27%
- Vitamin D 4%
- Vitamin E 10%
- Riboflavin 20%
- Niacin 7%
- Folate 19%
- Vitamin B-6 15%
- Vitamin B-12 12%
- Iron 14%

Spaghetti Squash Shrimp Scampi

Ingredients:

- 2.5 pounds of spaghetti squash cooking spray.
- ½ tablespoons unsalted butter
- ½ tablespoons olive oil teaspoon crushed red pepper
- 3 minced garlic cloves
- 8 ounces of peeled and deveined large raw shrimp
- 5 ounces of fresh baby spinach
- 3/8 teaspoon of kosher salt.
- Cooking Spray

How to Make:

1. Heat the oven to 375 degrees Fahrenheit, trim the ends of the spaghetti squash.
2. Cut spaghetti squash into 1 ½ rings while removing the seeds.
3. Spray metal tray rings with cooking spray.
4. Bake at 375 degrees Fahrenheit for 45 minutes
5. Let it cool.
6. Cut through each ring and open slightly to reach strands.
7. Carefully scrape out spaghetti-like squash strands.
8. Heat butter and oil on a pan/skillet at medium-high.
9. Add pepper and garlic, let it cook for 30 seconds, and stir.
10. Add shrimp and cook for 2 minutes

11. Add spinach and toss around until you see signs of wilting.

12. Finally, add the spaghetti squash strands and sprinkle some salt, then toss gently to combine. Now it's ready to be served.

Nutrition Facts:

- Per serving: 210 Calories
- 20 grams of Total Fat
- 7 grams of Saturated Fat
- 0 gram of Trans Fat
- 228 milligrams of Cholesterol
- 1544 milligrams of Sodium
- 10 grams of Total Carbohydrate
- 2 grams of Dietary Fibre
- 3 grams of Sugars
- 26 grams of Protein

Coffee-Rubbed Steak with Brussels Sprouts Salad

Ingredients:

- 1 tablespoon of ground coffee beans
- ¾ teaspoon of divided kosher salt
- ¾ teaspoon of divided black pepper
- 1 pound of hanger steak
- ¼ cup of divided olive oil
- 1 tablespoon of apple cider vinegar
- 2 teaspoons of Dijon mustard
- 1 teaspoon of honey
- 3 cups of shredded Brussels sprouts
- 1/3 cup of chopped toasted pecans
- 1 ounce of crumbled blue cheese

How to Make:

1. Heat a large on medium-high.
2. In a bowl, mix the coffee, 5/8 teaspoon salt, and ½ teaspoon of pepper in a small bowl.
3. Sprinkle the mixture on steak and press the mixture on the steak to adhere
4. Add 1 tablespoon of oil to the skillet.
5. Add steak and cook without moving until the bottom forms a crust for 3 minutes.

6. Turn steak over and cook until a thermometer insert-
ed in thickest portion registers 120 degrees Fahrenheit for 6 to 7 minutes, then turn off the heat.

7. Vinegar, honey mustard with remaining olive oil and
pepper and salt are to be whisked together in a large
bowl.

8. Add Brussels sprouts, pecan, and blue cheese, then
toss around for a good mix. Food is ready.

Nutritional Facts:

- Per serving: 427 Calories
- 31 grams of Total Fat
- 7 grams of Saturated Fat
- 21 grams of Unsaturated Fat
- 593 milligrams of Sodium
- 9 grams of Total Carbohydrates
- 4 grams of Dietary Fibre
- 3 grams of Sugar
- 29 grams of Protein
- 8% of Calcium
- Potassium 7%

Paleo Sushi Salmon Roll with Cauliflower Rice

Ingredients:

- 1 head of Cauliflower
- 1 tablespoon of Olive oil
- Sea salt
- 4 ounces of tuna
- 2 tablespoons of avocado mayonnaise
- 2 teaspoons of Sriracha
- 1 small cucumber
- ½ medium Avocado
- 2 sheets of nori
- Pickled ginger
- Wasabi
- Coconut aminos

How to Make:

1. Heat oven at 425 degrees Fahrenheit
2. Chop cauliflower into pieces small enough to be put in the food processor and blend each portion for 2 seconds.

3. Spread onto an aluminum foil-lined baking sheet and spray with olive oil.
4. Toast in oven for 30 minutes with occasional stirring.

5. Mince the tuna and mix with mayonnaise, sriracha, and salt.

6. Slice cucumber into strips (long recommended) and also slice the avocado into slices.

7. Put a piece of nor onto your towel/mat and cover with rice with a 1-inch gap at aside.

8. Place the topping on the opposite side of where the 1-inch gap is made.

9. Roll the sushi to the side with the gap and slice into 6 or 8 pieces.

10. Garnish with coconut amino, pickled ginger, and wasabi.

Nutrition Facts:

- 2 grams of Total Fat
- 440 milligrams of Protein
- 15 milligrams of Cholesterol
- 16 grams of Total Carbohydrates
- 1 gram of Dietary Fibre
- 4 grams of Sugar
- 7 grams of Protein
- 440 grams of Sodium

Orange, Tofu and Bell Pepper Stir-Fry

Ingredients:

- ¼ cup of divided canola oil
- 5 tablespoons of divided cornstarch
- 14 ounces of extra-firm water-packed tofu that is drained and cut into 3 to 4 inches in shapes of cubes
- ½ cup of fresh orange juice
- 1 cup of thinly sliced yellow onion
- 1 cup of sliced green bell pepper
- 1 cup of sliced red bell pepper
- 1 tablespoon thinly sliced garlic
- ½ teaspoon of grated (shredded) orange rind
- ½ teaspoon of crushed red pepper
- 3 tablespoons of reduced-sodium soy sauce
- 1 tablespoon of unseasoned rice vinegar
- 1 teaspoon light brown sugar
- ½ teaspoon kosher salt
- 2 of 8.8 ounces of precooked brown rice

How to Make:

1. Add 3 tablespoons of oil into a skillet/pan (one that doesn't stick) and cook at medium high.
2. Add ¼ cup of cornstarch and tofu in a bowl.

3. Add tofu to a pan and cook for 8 minutes, then remove tofu from pan.

4. Add remaining cornstarch and orange juice to a small bowl and mix.

5. Heat the remaining oil in a pan at medium high.

6. Add onion and bell peppers to a pan and cook for 5 minutes, then add garlic, orange rind, and crushed red pepper and cook for one minute.

7. Add the mixture from earlier in the bowl with the orange juice and cornstarch to the pan and boil.

8. Arrange plates, and each plate must have ½ cup of rice.

9. Stir tofu then add the toppings of tofu and cilantro sprinkles.

Nutrition Facts:

- Per serving: 219 Calories
- 555 milligrams of Sodium
- 8 grams of Total Fat
- 25 grams of Total Carbohydrates
- 1 gram of Dietary Fibre
- 17 grams of Sugars
- 11 grams of Protein
- Vitamin A 23%
- Vitamin C 108%
- Calcium 8%
- Iron 11%

Creamy Tomato Soup with Parmesan Crisps

Ingredients:

- ¼ cup of extra-virgin olive oil
- ¾ cup of chopped onion
- 1/3 cup of chopped carrot
- 6 large crushed garlic cloves
- 2 tablespoons of tomato paste
- 15 ounces of cans unsalted fire-roasted tomatoes
- 1 cup of organic vegetable broth
- 1/3 cup of half-and-half
- 3/8 teaspoon of kosher salt
- ½ cup of whole-wheat panko
- 2 ounces of shredded Parmigiano-Reggiano cheese
- ½ teaspoon of paprika
- ¼ teaspoon ground cumin
- 1/8 teaspoon ground red pepper

How to Make:

1. At medium high, heat the olive oil on a large saucepan.

2. Put onion, carrot, and garlic and cook for 5 minutes.

3. Apply tomato paste, tomatoes, and broth.

4. When it simmers, cook for an extra 6 minutes.

5. Stir in half-and-half and salt

6. Pour the mixture into a blender and blend it for about 30 seconds, and the recipe is done.

Nutrition Facts:

- Per serving: 326 Calories
- 20 grams of Total Fat
- 6 grams of Saturated Fat
- 14 grams of Unsaturated Fat
- 653 milligrams of Sodium
- 28 grams of Carbohydrates
- 4 grams of Fibre
- 11 grams of Sugars
- Calcium 16%
- Potassium 7%

Crispy Tuna Cakes

Ingredients:

- ½ cup of old-fashioned rolled oats
- 1 large egg, lightly beaten
- 2.6 ounces of pouch solid white tuna in water
- 1 teaspoon Dijon mustard
- 2 teaspoons fresh chopped parsley (optional to add later for garnish)
- ½ teaspoon of grated lemon rind
- 1/8 teaspoon of kosher salt
- 1/8 teaspoon freshly ground black pepper
- ¼ teaspoon garlic powder
- 2 teaspoons olive oil
- 2 cups arugula
- 2 tablespoons divided fresh lemon juice
- 1 tablespoon humus

How to Make:

1. Put the oats in the food processor and pulse for 10 seconds then add it to a bowl.

2. Mix in egg, tuna, mustard, w teaspoons of parsley, lemon rind, salt, pepper, and garlic powder.

3. Fill a 1/3 cup of the dry measuring cup with tuna mixture. Invert onto work surface; gently pat into a ¾-inch-thick patty.

4. Repeat with the remaining tuna mixture.

5. Now, heat the oil in a large pan/skillet at medium.

6. Add tuna cakes to the pan/skillet and cook for 3 to 4 minutes on each side.

7. Arrange arugula on a plate and mix with 1 tablespoon of lemon juice.

8. Serve with chopped fresh parsley (optional).

Nutrition Facts:

- Per serving: 423 Calories
- 20 grams of Total Fat
- 4 grams of Saturated Fat
- 614 milligrams of Sodium
- 33 grams of Total Carbohydrates
- 6 grams of Dietary Fibre
- 2 grams of Sugar
- 30 grams of Protein
- Calcium 9%

Chicken Meatball and Vegetable Soup

Ingredients:

- Cooking spray
- ½ pounds of ground chicken
- 2/3 of cup panko (Japanese breadcrumbs)
- 1 teaspoon of divided kosher salt
- 1 teaspoon of dried oregano
- 3 ounces of Parmesan cheese, grated and divided (about ¾ cup)
- 1 medium shredded garlic clove
- 2 tablespoons of canola oil
- 3 cups of sliced carrot
- 2 cups of chopped white onion
- ½ cups of diced celery
- 8 cups of unsalted of chicken stock
- 1 teaspoon freshly ground black pepper
- 2 bay leaves
- 12 ounces of fresh baby spinach

How to Make:

- Heat oven to 400 degrees Fahrenheit beforehand.
- Place a foil on a metal tray and coat with cooking spray.

- Add and mix chicken, panko, ¼ teaspoon salt, oregano, half of the cheese, garlic, and egg.

- Shape them into meatballs (2 tablespoons each), then put the meatballs in a pan with the heat set to 400 degrees Fahrenheit for 15 minutes.

- Increase the heat to high to boil for 2 to 3 minutes (until the meatballs have turned slightly to brown).

- Meanwhile, heat the oven to medium heat and add carrot, onion, and celery. Cook for 10 minutes while stirring.

- Add and mix stock, pepper bay leaves, and remaining ¾ teaspoon salt **in the pan**.

- Broil then reduce heat and let it simmer for 15 minutes.

- Add and stir the spinach in the pan.

- When the meatballs are ready, add them to the pan

- Turn off heat and stir in the meatballs, afterward sprinkle cheese on it. Now it's ready.

Nutrition Facts:

- Per serving: 190 Calories

- 2.8 grams of Total Fat

- 0.7 grams of Saturated Fat

- 0.7 grams of Polyunsaturated Fat

- 0.8 grams of Monounsaturated Fat

- 102.2 milligrams of Cholesterol

- 344.7 milligrams of Sodium

- 656.1 milligrams of Potassium

- 10.6 grams of Total Carbohydrate

- 2.3 grams of Dietary Fibre
- 2 grams of Sugars
- 28.3 grams of Protein
- Vitamin A 16.6%
- Vitamin B-12 .1%
- Vitamin B-6 30.9%
- Vitamin C 10.7%
- Vitamin D 2.5%
- Vitamin E 1.9%
- Calcium 4.2%
- Copper 4.3%
- Folate 10.4%
- Iron 10.8%
- Magnesium 10.2%
- Manganese 9.9%
- Niacin 55.9%
- Pantothenic Acid 9.0%
- Phosphorus 24.1%
- Riboflavin 10.2%
- Selenium 27.6%
- Thiamin 7.7%
- Zinc 7.6%

Stuffed Zucchini Boats

Ingredients:

- 4 large zucchinis (3 pounds)
- Cooking spray
- 1 cup of chopped onion
- 8 ounces of hot turkey Italian sausage
- 3/8 teaspoon divided kosher salt
- ½ ounces of small pieces of whole-grain
- 5 ounces of small and divided pieces of fresh mozzarella cheese
- 2 ½ teaspoons of divided olive oil
- 2 cups of halved cherry tomatoes
- ¼ of sliced basil (recommended to be sliced in a thin form)

How to Make:

1. Before starting, Heat the broiler at high.

2. Get 2 cups of zucchini pulp by removing it from the shell and applying them in a bowl (one that can be used for microwave purposes.

3. Cover with plastic, place the zucchini halves (shells) in the microwave and set microwave at high for 4 minutes

4. Heat a large pan on medium-high heat, then coat the pan with cooking spray.

5. Add onion and sausage to a pan and stir (recommended that the stirring crumble the sausage).

6. Add the zucchini pulp to the pan, and the zucchini halves on a **jelly-roll pan**.

7. Add ¼ teaspoon of salt to the first pan, then pour the mixture into the zucchini halves.

8. Blend bread in a food processor (until all that remains of the bread are crumbs).

9. Add 2 ounces of cheese and teaspoon oil and blend them in as well.

10. Broil 1 to 2 minutes (until the cheese melts and the crumbs show color change; brown).

11. When done add the bread cheese mix as toppings to the zucchini halves (shells)

12. With the remaining, mix the 3 ounces of cheese, tomatoes, basil, remaining 1/8 teaspoon salt, remaining 1 ½ teaspoon of oil, vinegar, and pepper in a small bowl, then pour the mixture on the zucchini halves. Now ready to be served.

Nutrition Facts:

- Per serving: 216.3 Calories
- 8.8 grams of Total Fat
- 46 milligrams of Cholesterol
- 487 milligrams of Sodium
- 7.4 grams of Total Carbs
- 1.9 grams of Dietary Fibre
- 23.8 grams of Protein

Low-Carb Beanless Chili

Ingredients:

- 2 tablespoons of olive oil
- 2 cups of fresh corn kernels
- 1 large chopped yellow onion
- 1 large chopped red bell pepper
- 2 medium chopped poblano chilies
- 1 tablespoon of chopped jalapeño chili
- 1 tablespoon of chopped garlic
- 16 ounces of round lean ground beef
- 2 tablespoons of tomato paste (the ones with no salt)
- 1 tablespoon of adobo sauce
- 1 tablespoon of dark chili powder
- 2 teaspoons dried oregano
- 15 ounces of canned tomato sauce (one with no salt)
- 14.5 ounces of canned diced tomatoes (the one with no salt)
- 1 cup of unsalted chicken stock
- ¼ teaspoon of kosher salt
- 1 tablespoon of fresh lime juice
- 1 large ripe avocado
- Some sliced fresh cilantro leaves lime wedges (as much as needed)

How to Make:

1. Before starting, heat the Dutch oven a medium high.

2. Add, stir, and cook the corn, onion, red bell pepper, poblano, jalapeño in the oven for about 10 minutes. (Stir only from time to time).

3. Add ground beef and cook for 7 minutes (until beef is crumbled).

4. Add tomato paste, adobe sauce, cumin, chili powder, and oregano and cook and stir for 1 minute.

5. Add tomato sauce, diced tomatoes, chicken stock, and salt.

6. Boil at a high temperature then brings to a simmer setting the oven to medium low for 20 minutes. (Stir from time to time).

7. Turn off heat.

8. Add lime juice and stir it in the mix.

9. After that, divide the chili into 6 bowls and toppings of avocado slices. Now it is ready to be served (optional to garnish with cilantro leaves and lime wedges).

Nutrition Facts:

- Per serving: 325 Calories

- 17 grams of Total Fat

- 6 grams of Saturated Fat

- 87 milligrams of Cholesterol

- 404 milligrams of Sodium

- 232 milligrams of Potassium

- 14 grams of Total Carbohydrates

- 2 grams of Dietary Fibre
- 6 grams of Sugar
- 27 grams of Protein
- Vitamin A 12%
- Vitamin C 37%
- Calcium 14%
- Iron 18%

Pistachio-Crusted Pork Cutlets

Ingredients:

- 4 ounces of pork cutlets
- ½ teaspoon of kosher salt
- ½ teaspoon of black pepper
- ¼ cup of cornstarch
- 1 large beaten egg
- 1 tablespoon of water
- ¾ cup of chopped roasted salted pistachios
- 2 tablespoons chopped fresh rosemary
- 2 tablespoons divided olive oil
- 1/8 teaspoon cayenne pepper
- 4 cups of arugula
- 2 tablespoons of lemon juice

How to Make:

1. Sprinkle kosher salt and black pepper on pork cutlets and let the cutlets soak in the cornstarch.

2. In a bowl, add egg and water and dip in the cutlets.

3. Then add roasted salted pistachios and rosemary to coat the cutlets.

4. Heat 1 tablespoon of olive oil and cayenne pepper in a pan/skillet.

5. Add the cutlets to the pan and cook for 3 minutes on each side (until the color of the cutlets changes to brown).

6. Add arugula, lemon juice, and 1 tablespoon of olive oil in a bowl.

7. Take out the cutlets and serve with the bowl of salad.

Nutrition Facts:

- Per serving 399 Calories
- 25 grams of Total Fat
- 5 grams of Saturated Fat
- 18 grams of Monounsaturated Fat
- 421 milligrams of Sodium
- 16 grams of Total Carbohydrates
- 3 grams of Dietary Fibre
- 3 grams of Sugar
- Calcium 12%

Spice-Roasted Salmon with Roasted Cauliflower

Ingredients:

- 1 tablespoon of olive oil
- 1 teaspoon of divided ground cumin
- ¾ teaspoon divided kosher salt
- 1/8 teaspoon freshly ground black pepper
- 4 cups cauliflower florets
- ¼ cup of chopped fresh cilantro
- ¼ cup golden raisins
- 1 tablespoon of fresh lemon juice
- ½ teaspoon of ground coriander
- 1/8 teaspoon of ground allspice
- 4 ½ ounces of salmon fillets (with skin on and about 1 inch thick)
- Cooking spray
- 4 lemon wedges

How to Make

1. Before starting, heat the oven to 450 degrees Fahrenheit.

2. In a large bowl, add olive oil, ½ teaspoon ground cumin, ¼ teaspoon of salt, and black pepper and mix in cauliflower florets (for coating the cauliflower).

3. On a metal tray, place the cauliflower and bake for 18 to 20 minutes at a temperature of 450 degrees Fahrenheit (until the cauliflower is brown and soft).

4. Now use the mixture to coat the cauliflower that was recently baked. Now it's ready to be served.

Nutrition Facts:

- Per serving: 270 Calories
- 11 grams of Total Fat
- 2 grams of Saturated Fat
- 8 grams of Polyunsaturated Fat
- 455 milligrams of Sodium
- 840 milligrams of Potassium
- Calcium 5%

Flax-Boosted Meatloaf

Ingredients:

- ½ cup of grated onion
- ¼ cup of the ground of flaxseed
- ½ teaspoon of kosher salt
- ½ teaspoon of black pepper
- 1 pound of 90% lean ground sirloin
- 1 shredded garlic clove
- 1 large egg
- 1/3 cup of organic ketchup
- Cooking spray

How to Make:

1. Before starting, heat the oven to 375 degrees Fahrenheit.

2. Mix egg, shredded garlic ground sirloin pepper, salt, ground flaxseed, and onion in a large bowl.

3. Spray cooking spray on a metal tray and line a foil on the tray.

4. Shape the mixture to an 8 by 4-inch loaf on the tray and add **organic** ketchup on the loaf.

5. Bake at 375 degrees Fahrenheit for 40 minutes.

6. When it's done, cut the meatloaf into 8 slices. The meal is ready.

Nutrition Facts:

- Per serving: 291 Calories
- 16 grams of Total Fat

- 5 grams of Saturated Fat
- 589 milligrams of Sodium
- 11 grams of Carbohydrates
- 2 grams of Dietary Fibre
- 6 grams of Sugar
- 26 grams of Protein
- Calcium 5%

Brown Sugar-Grilled Salmon with Zucchini and Fennel "Noodles"

Ingredients:

- Cooking spray
- 4 6 ounces of salmon fillets
- ¾ teaspoon of kosher salt
- 5/8 teaspoon of freshly divided ground black pepper
- 3 tablespoons of dark brown sugar
- 1 (12 ounces of) large peeled zucchini
- 1 small cored and sliced fennel bulb (thin)
- 1 tablespoon of chopped fresh dill
- 2 teaspoons of shredded orange rind
- ¼ cup of fresh orange juice
- 2 teaspoons of fresh lemon juice

How to Make:

1. Before starting, heat grill to medium-high, then coat with cooking spray.

2. On a flat surface, place fillets and sprinkle ¼ teaspoon of salt and ¼ teaspoon of pepper, then rub fillets with brown sugar.

3. Arrange fillets on the grill for 3 minutes on each side.

4. Turn off heat and use a vegetable peeler to shape zucchini into ribbons.

5. Add ½ teaspoon of salt in the remaining 3/8 tea-spoon pepper, zucchini, fennel, dill, orange rind, and juices in 4 bowls (divide evenly).

6. Add the fillet as a topping, and now it's ready.

Nutrition Facts:

- Per serving: 325 Calories
- 10 grams of Total Fat
- 2 grams of Saturated Fat
- 3 grams of Polyunsaturated Fat
- 3 grams of Monounsaturated Fat
- 90 milligrams of Cholesterol
- 480 milligrams of Sodium
- 19 grams of Total Carbohydrates
- 13 grams of Sugars
- 38 grams of Protein

Quick Chicken Piccata

Ingredients:

- 8 skinless, boneless chicken thighs (about 1 ½ pound)
- ½ teaspoon of divided kosher salt
- ½ teaspoon of freshly ground black pepper.
- 3 tablespoons of olive oil
- ½ cup of dry white wine
- 2 tablespoons of drained capers
- 4 crushed garlic cloves
- 1 fresh thyme sprig
- ¾ cup of unsalted chicken stock
- ½ tablespoons of fresh lemon juice
- 1 tablespoon unsalted butter
- 2 tablespoons of chopped fresh flat-leaf parsley

How to Make:

1. Prepare a plate and sprinkle ¼ teaspoon of salt and all of the pepper on chicken.

2. Prepare pan with 1 tablespoon of oil, then and chicken to pan, and cook for 5 minutes on each side.

3. After that, add wine, garlic, and thyme to the pan and cook for 2 minutes.

4. Add remaining salt and oil and stock to the pan and boil

5. After the mixture comes to a boil, reduce heat medium, and cook for 8 minutes.

6. Turn off the heat, add lemon juice and butter and stir.

7. Sprinkle parsley on the dish. The dish is ready.

Nutrition Facts:

- Per serving: 321 Calories
- 18 grams of Total Fat
- 7 grams of Saturated Fat
- 224 milligrams of Sodium
- 259 milligrams of Potassium
- 87 milligrams of Cholesterol
- 8 grams of Total Carbohydrates
- 1 gram of Sugar
- 25 grams of Protein
- Vitamin A 9%
- Vitamin C 16%
- Calcium 3%
- Iron 14%

Cheesy Sausage, Broccoli, and Quinoa Casserole

Ingredients:

- 2 ½ cups of water
- 2 cups of rinsed and drained quinoa
- 1 ½ tablespoon of olive oil
- ½ cup of chopped yellow onion
- ½ cup of chopped carrots
- 4 4 ounces of chopped chicken sausage
- 6 cups of fresh chopped broccoli florets
- ½ cup of sharp shredded cheddar cheese
- ¼ cup of all-purpose flour
- 2 tablespoons of unsalted butter
- 3 cloves of minced garlic
- 2 cups of whole milk
- 2 cups of low-sodium chicken stock
- 1 cup and 2/3 cup of sharp shredded cheddar cheese
- ½ teaspoon of dried thyme
- ½ teaspoon of kosher salt
- ½ teaspoon of black pepper
- Pinch of red pepper flakes
- ½ cup of panko breadcrumbs

- 1/3 cup of shredded mozzarella cheese
- 3 quint casserole dish (13x9) inches
- Cooking spray

How to Make:

1. Before starting, heat the oven to 400 degrees Fahrenheit.

2. Prepare a large skillet with 1 tablespoon of olive oil and heat it over medium.

3. Add onion, carrot, and chicken sausage to the pan and cook for 5 to 7 minutes. (until the vegetables become soft and the sausage changes its color to brown).

4. While the mixture is being cooked, prepare a bowl (one that can be used in a microwave) with water and broccoli. Cover the bowl (with something transparent) and place it inside the microwave. Microwave it for 4 to 5 minutes (you will notice steam on the cover, which will help determine whether it's ready).

5. Drain the broccoli from the water it soaked and add it to a **separate** large bowl.

6. Take the mixture from the pan and pour it into the large bowl with the broccoli (leave some of the liquid mixtures on the pan for later use).

7. Add butter and garlic to the pan, mix with the liquid leftover and heat over medium cooking temperature until it the butter melts.

8. Add flour and whisk until flour no longer remains.

9. Add milk and chicken stock.

10. Bring to a simmer then cook and whisk for 2 to 4 minutes. (Mixture will look thick)

11. Add thyme, salt, pepper, and red pepper flakes into the pan and stir.

12. Add 1 cup of cheddar cheese, whisk to melt the cheese into the sauce.

13. Add cooked quinoa to a large mixing bowl with other cooked ingredients.

14. Prepare a casserole dish and spray it with non-stick cooking spray and add **½ of the mixture** in the pan to the dish (The remaining mixture in the pan can go in the fridge for a second meal 'up to 3 months !!'). Sprinkle ½ cup of cheddar cheese.

15. Add panko breadcrumbs, 2/3 cup of cheddar cheese, and 1/3 cup of mozzarella cheese to the mixture (now called a casserole) on the with remaining ½ teaspoon of olive oil.

16. Bake the mixture for 18 to 20 minutes (casserole will change color slightly to brown with bubbles formed).

Nutrition Facts:

- Per serving: 296 Calories
- 13 grams of Total Fat
- 5 grams of Saturated Fat
- 2 grams of Polyunsaturated Fat
- 399 milligrams of Sodium
- 48 milligrams of Cholesterol
- 28 grams of Total Carbohydrates
- 4 grams of Dietary Fibre
- 4 grams of Sugars
- 17 grams of Protein

Night Meals & Drinks

Carrot Juice

Ingredients:
- Carrots (as much as needed)
- 1 apple
- Half an orange
- Half a ginger

How to Make:
1. Prepare a blender and blend carrots.
2. (Optional) Add the rest of the optional ingredients for a detox drink.

Benefits:
- Burning Fat through bile secretion
- Maintain good eyesight
- Slows aging
- Prevents Cancer, Heart Disease, and Diabetes

Amla Juice

Ingredients:
- Amla (as much as needed)

How to Make:
1. Squeeze amlas into a cup/ Use a food processor to get the juice out of the amlas

- Accelerates metabolism (increases the rate at which your body changes)

Pomegranate Juice

Ingredients:
- Pomegranate (as much as needed)

How to Make:
- Use a food processor to make juice with the pomegranates.

Benefits:
- High fiber (which helps in burning fat).
- Excretes waste faster.

Karela Juice

Ingredients:
- Karela (as much as needed)

How to Make:
- Wash and chop the karelas.
- Prepare a blender and blend then chopped karelas.

Benefits:
- Stimulates the liver to secrete acids (Increase Metabolism).

Pineapple Juice

Ingredients:
- Pineapple (as much as needed)

How to Make:

- Skin and chop pineapples.

- Prepare a blender and blend the chopped pineapples.

Benefits:

- Burns away excess stomach fat

WaterMelon Juice

Ingredients:

- Watermelon

How to Make:

- Chop and skin watermelon.

- Blend in a blender.

Benefits:

- Helps burn fat

Nuts, Walnuts, Almonds

Ingredients:

- Any of the above-mentioned

How to Make:

- Prepare a bowl and pour in the ingredients.

Benefits:

- Burns fat to digest these.

CONCLUSION

In the end, most foods are beneficial if taken the right way. It is also good to combine foods to get the ultimate nutrient supply. As necessary as our necessities are to get through the day with a satisfied tummy, a wrong choice in diet can lead us down a long wrong path that can lead to severe injuries, whether as a rookie with little information or as a fast-food lover with craving to quench. In this book, you learned how to make healthy while being tasty, which is excellent for beginners like you. Remember to regulate your intake of risky fruits and vegetables, especially acidic ones.

FINAL WORDS

Thank you again for purchasing this book!

We really hope this book is able to help you.

The next step is for you to **join our email newsletter** to receive updates on any upcoming new book releases or promotions. You can sign up for free and as a bonus, you will also receive our "*7 Fitness Mistakes You Don't Know You're Making*" book! This bonus book breaks down many of the most common fitness mistakes and will demystify many of the complexities and science of getting into shape. Having all this fitness knowledge and science organized into an actionable step-by-step book will help you get started in the right direction in your fitness journey! To join our free email newsletter and grab your free book, please visit the link and sign up: **www.effingopublishing.com/gift**

Finally, if you enjoyed this book, then we would like to ask you for a favor, would you be kind enough to leave a review for this book? It would be greatly appreciated! Thank you and good luck in your journey!

About the Co-Authors

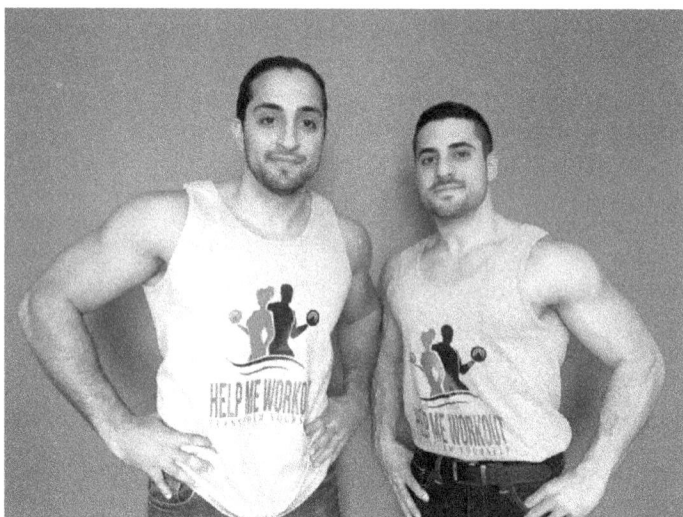

Our name is Alex & George Kaplo; we're both certified personal trainers from Montreal, Canada. Will start off by saying we are not the biggest guys you will ever meet and this has never really been our goal. In fact, we started working out to overcome our biggest insecurity when we were younger, which was our self-confidence. You may be going through some challenges right now, or you may simply want to get fit, and we can certainly relate.

For us personally, we always kind were interested in the

health & fitness world and wanted to gain some muscle due to the numerous bullying in our teenage years. We figured we can do something about how our body looks like. This was the beginning of our transformation journey. We had no idea where to start, but we both just got started. We felt worried and afraid at times that other people would make fun of us for doing the exercises the wrong way. We always wished we had a friend to guide us and who could just show us the ropes.

After a lot of work, studying and countless trial and errors. Some people began to notice how we were both getting more fit and how we were starting to form a keen interest in the topic. This led many friends and new faces to come to us and ask us for fitness advice. At first, it seemed odd when people asked us to help them get in shape. But what kept us going is when they started to see changes in their own body and told us it's the first time that they saw real results! From there, more people kept coming to us, and it made both of us realize after so much reading and studying in this field that it did help us but it also allowed us to help others. To date, we have coached and trained numerous clients who have achieved some pretty amazing results.

Today, both of us own & operate this publishing business, where we bring passionate and expert authors to write about health and fitness topics. We also run an online fitness business and we would love to connect with you by inviting you to visit the website on the following page and signing up to our e-mail newsletter (you will even get a free book).

Last but not least, if you are in the position we were once in and you want some guidance, don't hesitate and ask... will be there to help you out!

Your coaches,

Alex & George Kaplo

Download another book for Free

We want to thank you for purchasing this book and offer you another book (just as long and valuable as this book), "Health & Fitness Mistakes You Don't Know You're Making", completely free.

Visit the link below to sign up and receive it:

www.effingopublishing.com/gift

In this book, we will break down the most common health & fitness mistakes, you are probably committing right now, and will reveal how you can easily get in the best shape of your life!

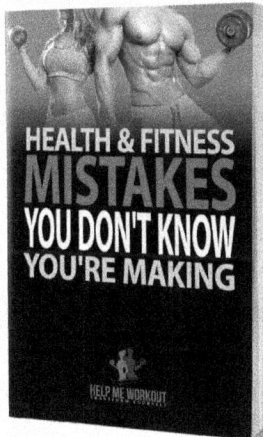

In addition to this valuable gift, you will also have an opportunity to get our new books for free, enter giveaways, and receive other valuable emails from us. Again, visit the link to sign up:

www.effingopublishing.com/gift

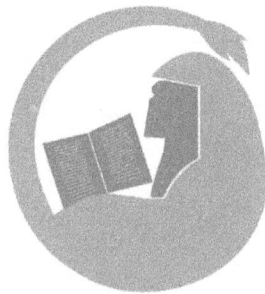

EFFINGO
Publishing

For more great books visit:

EffingoPublishing.com

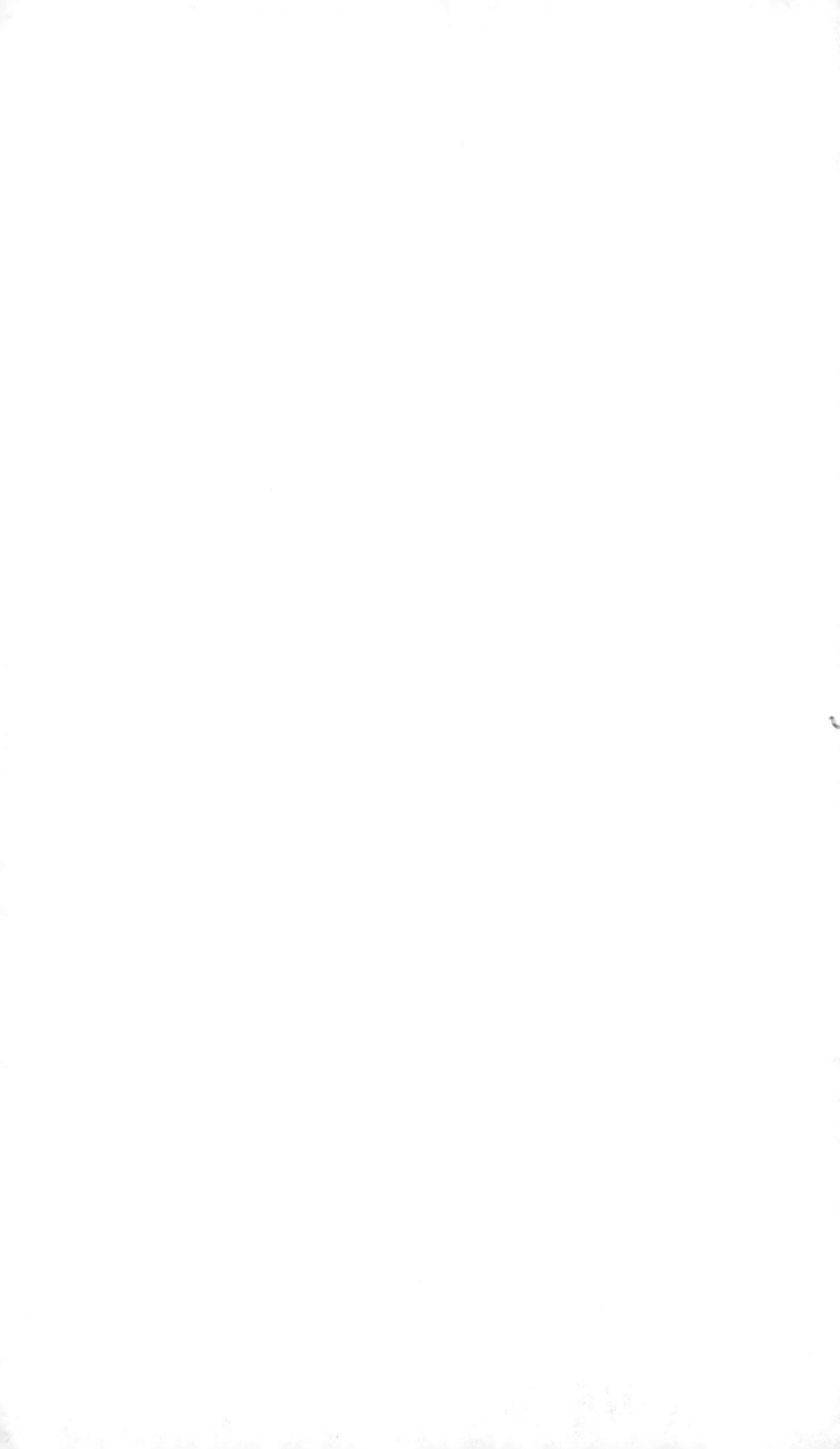